Movement Disorders

SECOND EDITION

Richard A. Walsh, MB, MD, MRCPI
Clinical Senior Lecturer in Neurology
Trinity College Dublin
Tallaght Hospital
Dublin, Ireland

Robertus M. A. de Bie, MD, PhD
Professor of Neurology
University of Amsterdam
Academic Medical Center
Amsterdam, Netherlands

Susan H. Fox, MBChB, MRCP(UK), PhD
Associate Professor Neurology
University of Toronto
Toronto Western Hospital
Toronto, Canada

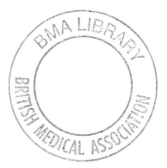

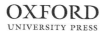

OXFORD
UNIVERSITY PRESS

OXFORD
UNIVERSITY PRESS

Oxford University Press is a department of the University of Oxford. It furthers
the University's objective of excellence in research, scholarship, and education
by publishing worldwide. Oxford is a registered trade mark of Oxford University
Press in the UK and certain other countries.

Published in the United States of America by Oxford University Press
198 Madison Avenue, New York, NY 10016, United States of America.

© Oxford University Press 2017

First Edition published in 2013
Second Edition published in 2017

Library of Congress Cataloging-in-Publication Data
Names: Walsh, Richard A., 1978- , author. | Bie, Robertus M. A. de, author. | Fox, Susan H., author.
Title: Movement disorders / Richard A. Walsh, Robertus M.A. de Bie, Susan H. Fox.
Other titles: What do I do now?
Description: Second edition. | Oxford ; New York : Oxford University Press, [2017] |
Series: What do I do now? | Includes bibliographical references and index.
Identifiers: LCCN 2016014241 (print) | LCCN 2016014861 (ebook) |
ISBN 9780190607555 (pbk. : alk. paper) | ISBN 9780190607562 (e-book) |
ISBN 9780190607579 (e-book) | ISBN 9780190607586 (online)
Subjects: | MESH: Movement Disorders—diagnosis | Movement Disorders—therapy | Neurodegenerative
Diseases—complications | Neurodegenerative Diseases—therapy
Classification: LCC RC376.5 (print) | LCC RC376.5 (ebook) | NLM WL 390 | DDC 616.8/3—dc23
LC record available at https://lccn.loc.gov/2016014241

9 8 7 6 5 4 3 2 1

Printed by Webcom, Inc., Canada

Contents

Preface

In this second edition of *What Do I Do Now? Movement Disorders*, we have added 14 new chapters and updated others that appeared in the first edition. The field of movement disorders remains one of the most exciting subspecialties within neurology, with continued advances in our understanding of the genetic and pathological basis for these diseases. While attempting to include some new themes to reflect these changes, the focus remains almost entirely clinical, with a pragmatic and practical approach offering solutions to commonly encountered problems. As before, we have aimed to keep chapters short and accessible, with 'high yield' information presented in an informal, problem-solving manner.

This book is suitable for general neurologists, trainees in movement disorders, as well as community and hospital-based general physicians who will encounter many of the more common and some of the rarer presentations included in this edition. Information provided is digestible and equally amenable to being carried in a white coat or used as a ready reference text in the clinic or office. We hope each time you dip into a chapter you come away with a clinical pearl or nugget that enhances your knowledge and your practice.

Contributors

Marina Picillo, MD
Researcher, Center for
Neurodegenerative Diseases
Department of Medicine and
Surgery, Neuroscience section
University of Salerno
Salerno, Italy

Susanne E. M. Ten Holter, MD
Department of Neurology
Medical Centre Haaglanden
The Hague, The Netherlands

PART I

Parkinson's Disease

1 Smoothing out the Ups and Downs

Richard A. Walsh

You are reviewing a 63-year-old man with a diagnosis of idiopathic Parkinson's disease of 10 years' duration, treated for 8 years. He has had a relatively uncomplicated course to date, continuing to work at a bank, with no cognitive complaints and good tolerance of the dopamine agonist you had started him on 7 years ago. Four years ago, you added low-dose levodopa due to progression of his tremor that had become a nuisance at work, where colleagues, unaware of his condition, had commented on it. It had failed to respond to increasing doses of ropinirole. He is currently taking 18 mg ropinirole once daily and levodopa–carbidopa 100 mg/25 mg four times daily. He reports continued good "on" time where he feels he moves normally. His only new complaints are increasing weight, often snacking throughout the day, and a return of the right upper limb tremor 30 minutes predose. He is unaware of dyskinesia, but you note some mild dyskinetic movement of his right foot when animated.

What do you do now?

INITIAL MEDICAL MANAGEMENT OF MOTOR FLUCTUATIONS IN PARKINSON'S DISEASE

It is sometimes helpful to use the analogy of a game of chess when explaining the approach to managing the motor complications of Parkinson's disease to newly diagnosed patients. I describe how the disease can be expected to change slowly as time goes on and the aim of the physician to outmaneuver it by being a few moves ahead at all times. We know this is possible because the emergence of motor complications tends to be reasonably predictable and almost an inevitability as years on therapy pass by. The analogy can be useful in helping patients understand the complexity and dynamic nature of their disease as well as preparing them for what will be many years of regular medication adjustments. This explanation can even be reassuring to patients who like to believe their doctor knows what to expect and has a number of treatment options to introduce when needed in the future.

THE THREE STAGES OF PARKINSON'S DISEASE

In simplistic terms, the natural history of the motor aspect of Parkinson's disease can be categorized into three main epochs, not all equal in duration:

1. The so-called "honeymoon period" is when motor symptoms respond well to dopaminergic therapy, allowing many patients to feel close to normal for much, if not all, of their day. This phase often includes treatment with a dopamine agonist in monotherapy but also the early stages of levodopa therapy in which the "long-duration effect" allows the benefit from individual doses to merge seamlessly together. This phenomenon is due to the buffering effect of surviving nigral neurons, which take up ingested levodopa and store it for later use well beyond its 90-minute plasma half-life.

2. After 5 or more years of levodopa therapy, most patients will experience motor complications, typically beginning with an awareness that the benefit of the first of three daily doses has faded by the time the next dose is due. This "wearing off" is characterized by a re-emergence of previously well-controlled symptoms. Dyskinesia may also be noticed for the first time, initially as subtle and nonbothersome choreiform movements, often unnoticed by the patient. Dyskinesia can be expected in 50% of patients after 5 years of levodopa therapy. A spouse may report a tendency to rock back and forth or dyskinetic neck movements coinciding with the peak effect of each or some doses of levodopa.

3. "Advanced" Parkinson's disease is a term sometimes used to describe patients who have had many years of disease and for whom motor complications (on–off fluctuations and troublesome dyskinesia) have become a prominent and constant problem. Patients in this stage of disease often have additional nonmotor and levodopa-unresponsive complications such as dementia and postural instability. The nondisabling wearing-off experienced in the earlier stages is replaced by sudden and unpredictable "off" periods, dose failures, delayed responses, and freezing. These severe motor fluctuations can leave patients experiencing brief islands of relatively good movement in a day otherwise marked by hours of disabling "off" time in which freezing, akinesia, and tremor can leave them fully dependent.

PRINCIPLES TO GUIDE MANAGEMENT OF MOTOR FLUCTUATIONS

Listen to the Patient to Allow Treatment to Be Titrated to the Patient's Movement Requirements

A 40-year-old professional golfer with early onset Parkinson's disease will have very different expectations and requirements compared to an 80-year-old nursing home resident. This is not to imply that the older patient's needs are less important; however, for a patient largely confined to a chair or bed, the re-emergence of a moderate tremor for 1 hour before each dose may be tolerated, whereas in the golfer it clearly would not. It is also important not to change treatment just because you can do so. I always ask patients, "Would you be happy if I said your last week would reflect how you are likely to function for the next 12 months?" If they are broadly happy with this notion, I tend not to tinker with their pills for the sake of it. If they believe they have daily symptoms that adversely affect function on a social, professional, or recreational level, then I believe there is good rationale for a change.

Take the Time to Get an Accurate Picture of a Typical Day

When first questioned about their motor performance, patients with Parkinson's disease will often explain how yesterday was particularly bad or how their morning dose prior to clinic did not work as well as expected and provide their own interpretation of why this was the case. These are important issues for them of course, but isolated fluctuations may not always be representative of the larger picture. While acknowledging that day-to-day fluctuations occur, emphasize that what you need is an *average* picture of their day. With some help, most patients will be able to provide a good outline of how long their "on" response tends to last with each dose and for what proportion of the day they are bothered by dyskinesia. With this information taken in a patient manner, it is far easier to make treatment changes. There will always be patients for whom motor fluctuations are so unpredictable that it is impossible for them to give a broad overview, and managing these patients can present a particular challenge. In the future, there will likely be increased use of automated technology that patients can wear on a wrist to give an automated and objective assessment of bradykinesia and dyskinesia.

Know When Less Is More

For the first 10–15 years of disease, the symptoms of Parkinson's disease are managed by the addition and layering of dopaminergic agents and enzyme inhibitors in an attempt to deliver a steady state of performance. Many patients will be treated with adjuvant agents such as anticholinergic drugs or amantadine for dyskinesia. As the condition progresses with an accumulation of cortical disease and the emergence of hallucinations and cognitive impairment, a measured retreat is often necessary to minimize side effects. Anticholinergics and amantadine are particularly poorly tolerated in patients older than age 70 years, and the improvement in what was believed to be disease-related cognitive decline can sometimes be dramatic once they are slowly withdrawn.

STRATEGIES FOR THE SECOND STAGE WHEN MOTOR COMPLICATIONS EMERGE

Motor fluctuations will not typically emerge for patients maintained on a dopamine agonist or monoamine oxidase B (MAO-B) inhibitor in monotherapy, or indeed in combination. As time progresses, the tendency is for additional dopaminergic therapies to be layered on to achieve an adequate motor response, and there are a number of options (Table 1.1) Ultimately, as was the case in this patient, it becomes necessary to add in levodopa when these less potent agents are not sufficient to manage symptoms or when side effects make dose increases a less attractive choice. Levodopa is typically started on a three-times-daily regimen, but over time the long-duration effect wanes, bringing on the wearing-off phenomenon. This early tailing off of individual levodopa doses can be managed by increasing the dose of a longer acting dopamine agonist being used or addition of a once-daily MAO-B inhibitor if not already in place. If these options are not available or not tolerated due to

TABLE 1.1 **Treatment Options for the Management of Motor Symptoms in Parkinson's Disease**

	Advantages	*Disadvantages*
MAO-B inhibitors Selegiline Rasagiline	Once-daily drugs Generally well tolerated	Small overall symptomatic response Selegiline can cause sleep disturbance, particularly when taken late in the day
Dopamine agonists Ropinirole Pramipexole Rotigotine	Available in once-daily or patch formulations, improving convenience and compliance Very low incidence of dyskinesia in monotherapy Can provide adequate symptom relief in monotherapy	Impulse control disorders are an increasingly recognized side effect Contribute to cognitive impairment and hallucinations in older patients Inevitably need bolstering with levodopa with disease progression
Levodopa/carbidopa	Most effective oral agent for symptom control Generally better tolerated than all other options	Contributes to genesis of dyskinesia Short-acting drug; multiple doses required with advancing disease Can also cause impulse control disorders and a greater cause of punding than dopamine agonists
COMT inhibitors Entacapone Tolcapone	Useful for maintaining duration of motor response with levodopa Generally well tolerated Available in compound preparation with levodopa	Can worsen previously nonbothersome dyskinesia Potential hepatotoxicity with tolcapone
Amantadine	Useful for reducing dyskinesia Mild antiparkinsonian effect, useful for some levodopa refractory tremor Worth trying for intractable freezing of gait	Poorly tolerated over the age of 65 years Commonly contributes to hallucinations
Anticholinergics	Can help otherwise refractory tremor	Poorly tolerated in older patients

side effects, a catechol-*O*-methyltransferase (COMT) inhibitor (entacapone, 200 mg with each levodopa dose) can be added. Tolcapone, an alternative COMT inhibitor, is available in some countries and requires strict monitoring of hepatic function. The addition of a COMT inhibitor will also have the effect of increasing the peak effect of levodopa, which can produce or exacerbate dyskinesia. If these options are already exhausted, a reduction of the interdose interval can be a simple way to attack wearing off, albeit with the added inconvenience of having to remember to take an extra dose.

APPROACH IN THIS CASE

As described previously, this patient has had a predictable emergence of early motor fluctuations with wearing off that is, although mild, troublesome in his opinion. He continues to work and would like to avoid visible manifestations of his Parkinson's disease, in the form of either dyskinesia or tremor. It is important to take note of the weight gain because this suggests a possible impulse control disorder as a complication of his dopamine agonist, which he is taking at a reasonably high dose. He is on a four-times-daily regimen, giving him a 4-hour interval between doses at 7 a.m., 11 a.m., 3 p.m., and 7 p.m. The final point to note is the evident dyskinesia, which is not an issue for him currently but must be taken into consideration when making a treatment change.

My instinct here would be to avoid pushing the dopamine agonist higher. The tremor had failed to respond to increasing doses in the past and is therefore unlikely to respond now. Increasing doses of dopamine agonists can often demonstrate a law of diminishing marginal returns, with only increasing side effects as you move upward from moderate to high doses. On this note, this patient has already demonstrated some impulse control disorder features that will undoubtedly worsen with higher agonist doses.

A simple move would be to change interdose interval from 4 to 3 or 3.5 hours. This will make his regimen more complicated and does often have the effect of increasing peak dose dyskinesia, particularly toward the end of the day when there tends to be a cumulative effect of levodopa ingested earlier in the day. The addition of a COMT inhibitor can prolong the effect of each dose, buying back approximately 1 hour of good "on" time each day. This is sometimes sufficient, but there is also often a tendency to increase peak dose dyskinesia. It is often suggested that individual doses of levodopa should be reduced by 20–30% to combat this effect, but in practice each dose of levodopa can only be halved on a practical level, which is an excessive reduction for the addition of a COMT inhibitor.

The best choice in this man may be the addition of rasagiline or selegiline. This step is often unavailable because of the fact that many patients are started on these agents at onset due to interest in their disease-modifying potential, although this is not evidence based. Addition for motor fluctuations is a conservative step that can also buy back approximately 1 hour of effective "on" time without running the risk of agonist-related side effects with less potential to exacerbate dyskinesia.

It is inevitable that this patient will need up to a five-times-daily regimen during the next 3 years, and as options to smooth out motor fluctuations are used up, advanced therapies may come into play. The goal of the current consultation, however, is to make a change that restores some function while avoiding side effects.

KEY POINTS TO REMEMBER

- Treatment in Parkinson's disease is not disease modifying, only symptomatic. Therefore, the aim should be to maximize symptom control when the patient believes he or she needs it and not just because you can do so.
- Parkinson's disease progresses slowly. Sudden deteriorations in function are typically due to extrinsic factors such as intercurrent illness and do not warrant a treatment change. When a patient gives a reasonably reliable picture of motor fluctuations that have a meaningful impact on quality of life, discuss a change of timing, dose, or drug.
- Not all wearing off, even where predictable, needs a change in treatment regimen. Many patients will report a re-emergence of symptoms that are neither bothersome nor disabling. Although the mantra is to smooth out dopaminergic stimulation, smoothing out every crease for the sake of making a change is not always a necessity.
- Dopamine agonists remain very useful agents for the management of mild to moderate parkinsonism in young to middle-aged patients. These agents can reduce the amount of levodopa required, acting as a levodopa-sparing agent. It is important to know when dopamine agonists are no longer effective in controlling symptoms or are causing unwanted side effects.

Further Reading

da Silva-Junior FP, Braga-Neto P, Sueli Monte F, de Bruin VM. Amantadine reduces the duration of levodopa-induced dyskinesia: A randomized, double-blind, placebo-controlled study. *Parkinsonism Relat Disord* 2005;11(7):449–452.

Hely MA, Reid WG, Adena MA, Halliday GM, Morris JG. The Sydney multicenter study of Parkinson's disease: The inevitability of dementia at 20 years. *Mov Disord* 2008;23(6):837–844.

Nutt JG. Motor fluctuations and dyskinesia in Parkinson's disease. *Parkinsonism Relat Disord* 2001;8(2):101–108.

Nutt JG, Carter JH, Woodward WR. Long-duration response to levodopa. *Neurology* 1995;45(8):1613–1616.

Rascol O, Fitzer-Attas CJ, Hauser R, et al. A double-blind, delayed-start trial of rasagiline in Parkinson's disease (the ADAGIO study): Prespecified and post-hoc analyses of the need for additional therapies, changes in UPDRS scores, and non-motor outcomes. *Lancet Neurol* 2011;10(5):415–423.

2   "He Wants It All the Time, Doctor"

Robertus M. A. de Bie

The patient is 57 years old and has had Parkinson's disease for 17 years. The disease started with slowness and stiffness on the right side. Nine years into the disease, he had right-sided symptoms only, though severe, and he underwent a left-sided pallidotomy. This was very effective. Over time, the symptoms worsened, and now he has medication-induced motor response fluctuations, dysarthria, and difficulty walking. He is referred for treatment with deep brain stimulation. Upon inquiry, it appeared that he experienced problems with gambling and hypersexuality during the past 7 years, but he denies this to be a problem. He takes levodopa/carbidopa 100/25 mg 5 tablets per day, levodopa/carbidopa sustained release 100/25 mg 12 tablets per day, selegiline 5 mg BID, entacapone 200 mg QID, amantadine 100 mg BID, and ropinirole extended release 24 mg per day. He initially visits you alone, without his wife.

What do you do now?

IMPULSE-CONTROL DISORDERS IN PARKINSON'S DISEASE

Parkinson's disease (PD) may be accompanied by impulse-control disorders such as pathological gambling, hypersexuality, compulsive shopping, and compulsive eating. Patients may also display addiction-like behavior toward taking levodopa, referred to as "dopamine dysregulation syndrome." Typically, patients with PD are not distressed by the behaviors associated with the impulse-control disorders, and the aberrant behaviors often go unnoticed because patients experience these as internally consistent with their thoughts and behaviors. From studies into the prevalence among patients who visit specialized PD clinics, it appears that pathological gambling occurs in 4% of patients. In patients who use dopamine agonists, the frequency is higher—up to 8%. The frequency of hypersexuality is 3–8%; that of compulsive shopping is almost 2%.

There is an individual susceptibility (hereditary and/or environmental) for impulse-control disorders within the framework of PD. Factors associated with a higher risk for impulse-control disorders are a young age at disease onset, a history of addictive behavior before the disease started, a family history of addiction such as alcoholism, and being male. In addition, there is a relationship with medication use, with dopamine agonists having the highest risk. The treatment of impulse-control disorders consists of lowering or stopping the dopamine agonist, treating any possible depression or anxiety disorder, and involving the family and spouse. Referral to a psychiatrist may be required. There are reports that impulse-control disorders disappeared following treatment with deep-brain stimulation of the subthalamic nucleus because the dopamine agonists were subsequently stopped.

Another behavioral disorder that may be seen in the context of PD is "punding." Punding is defined as complex, prolonged, aimless, and stereotyped behavior with a fascination for repetitive actions of, for example, machines, sorting and investigating ordinary objects (e.g., buttons, labels, and tools), grooming, hoarding, driving or walking around aimlessly, and elaborate monologues. Patients experience punding as disruptive and unproductive but appear to find it very unpleasant to be disturbed during the behavior.

If the patient and spouse recognize that the behavior is abnormal, they may not be aware that it could be due to the anti-PD medication. Frequently, patients have enormous debts or serious issues in their relationship before the treating physician knows about the problem and can try to help. Therefore, it is very important to inform every patient and spouse about impulse-control disorders, especially when the patient starts taking dopamine agonists. In particular, the clinician should ask the patient and especially the family members about any impulsive behavior.

In this case, we invited the patient to come to another appointment with his wife. She confirmed that he was hypersexual and that he made unreasonable and frequent demands. The patient did not believe that the hypersexuality was a problem. Five years ago, they had decided to live apart, but they had not told their adult children. Usually, the patient visited the neurologist alone. Once, he brought his wife and the hypersexuality was discussed. The neurologist advised him to reduce the dopamine agonist dosage (ropinirole). Subsequently, he continued to visit the neurologist on his own and denied any hypersexuality. The ropinirole dosage was increased again. We stopped the ropinirole, and he had a successful deep-brain stimulation treatment. To date, the hypersexuality did not recur.

KEY POINTS TO REMEMBER

- Inform the patient and spouse that impulse-control disorders are possible sequelae of the PD medication, especially the dopamine agonists.
- The impulse-control disorders occur commonly without subjective distress or are frequently hidden or go unnoticed because they are experienced as being internally consistent with the patient's thoughts.

Further Reading

Evans AH, Katzenschlager R, Paviour D, et al. Punding in Parkinson's disease: Its relation to the dopamine dysregulation syndrome. *Mov Disord* 2004;19(4):397–405 [includes a video].

Voon V, Fox SH. Medication-related impulse control and repetitive behaviors in Parkinson disease. *Arch Neurol* 2007;64(8):1089–1096.

Voon V, Potenza MN, Thomsen T. Medication-related impulse control and repetitive behaviors in Parkinson's disease. *Curr Opin Neurol* 2007;20:484–492.

3 Becoming a Little Forgetful

Susan H. Fox and Marina Picillo

A 69-year-old, retired engineer is referred with a 5-year history of Parkinson's disease (PD). At onset, he presented with gait impairment and slowness of movements most prevalent on the left side. After the diagnosis, he started taking levodopa with an excellent response. Nowadays, he is quite satisfied with his motor function, although he has mild motor fluctuations with predictable wearing off approximately 15 minutes before each dose. Both he and his wife, however, are concerned about his worsening cognitive abilities. He has difficulties in following a conversation or reading a book. His wife confirms he has always been a well-organized person, although now he struggles with planning. He reports a significant worsening of his mood that has been resistant to treatment with antidepressants. According to his wife, he used to be a very active man, whereas now he has become more passive and withdrawn. At night, he has had trouble sleeping and has had nightmares for many years, but recently he also started to have visual hallucinations when awake.

What do you do now?

COGNITIVE IMPAIRMENT IN PARKINSON'S DISEASE

The reported change in cognitive skills that manifest in daily life with difficulties in planning, a change in mood, and apathy all suggest early cognitive impairment in PD. In such individuals, ensuring the symptoms are not all due to depression is important, and help from psychiatry colleagues can be invaluable. Sleep disturbances may also exacerbate or cause apparent cognitive issues, and they need to be reviewed carefully. In addition, it is important to ensure that the symptoms are not associated with "off" periods because many people with PD report low mood and impaired thinking in low-dopamine states.

Cognitive impairment and dementia are common in PD and are associated with a more rapid motor and functional decline, increased mortality, increased caregiver burden, as well as being an independent risk factor for nursing home placement. In the 20-year follow-up of the Sydney Multicenter Study, 83% of survivors were affected by dementia, suggesting an inevitability in long-standing disease. A spectrum of cognitive dysfunction is observed in PD, with mild cognitive impairment (MCI) typically preceding dementia by several years.

This patient appears to be experiencing attentional and executive impairment (e.g., difficulties in concentration and planning activities), accompanied by behavioral symptoms such as depression and apathy. He is exhibiting well-formed visual hallucinations, which commonly accompany cognitive impairment, sometimes accompanied by delusions where insight is lost. In addition, he probably has rapid eye movement sleep behavior disorder, which is considered to be a risk factor for the development of dementia.

When a patient with an established diagnosis of PD presents with cognitive decline, the first step is a proper assessment of the nature and cause of cognitive impairment and associated behavioral symptoms. These symptoms may be the consequence of the natural course of the disease, as well as the result of other factors, such as adverse effects of drugs, systemic diseases (e.g., urinary tract infections), or metabolic problems (e.g., uncontrolled diabetes). Mode of onset and the course of symptoms, as well as the presence of systemic findings, should guide the approach to patients and drive further investigations. All medications, especially those recently introduced, and dose changes should be reviewed. Drugs that can potentially contribute to cognitive dysfunction, such as selegiline, amantadine, anticholinergics, tricyclic antidepressants, benzodiazepines, and dopamine agonists, should be gradually discontinued, generally in that order. Depression may significantly affect cognitive abilities and should be addressed with the appropriate expert input.

Once other causes have been excluded, the next step is to establish the degree of cognitive impairment and clarify if the patient is manifesting an overt dementia. The Montreal Cognitive Assessment (MoCA) is a quick and easy test to screen for early detection of cognitive deterioration in primary care settings (available at http://www.mocatest.org). It covers eight cognitive domains: short-term and delayed verbal memory, visuospatial abilities, executive functions, attention, concentration, working memory, language, and orientation to time and place. It has been reported that a cutoff less than 26 is appropriate when applying the test as a screening tool for PD-related dementia. A formal diagnosis of dementia can be established when cognitive impairment in more than one domain is severe enough to impair functional independence in the course of the component parts of daily living (social, occupational, or personal care). A failure to meet this benchmark could be consistent with a diagnosis of MCI, which is addressed in the next section. Asking the patient to describe his or her parkinsonian medication regimen has been proposed as a simple way to evaluate the impact of cognitive decline on daily life (e.g., "Are you still able to take the prescribed pills reliably?" or "Can you describe your medication regimen for me?"). Interviewing the caregiver is the most crucial step in establishing the functional independence of the patient at this stage.

MILD COGNITIVE IMPAIRMENT

In an attempt to standardize the definition of cognitive impairment in PD, a Movement Disorders Society (MDS) task force proposed diagnostic criteria for MCI, thereby defining a clinical syndrome analogous to MCI in Alzheimer's disease. The criteria are displayed in Box 3.1 and include additional recommendations in terms of neuropsychological testing and subtyping. Executive function represents the most common cognitive domain affected in PD, reflecting the dopaminergic dysfunction of the frontostriatal network. However, impairment in attention, explicit memory, and visuospatial function may be common as well and may have a nondopaminergic etiology (e.g., cholinergic dysfunction). The MDS PD MCI criteria provide a framework for domain-specific subtyping by number (single vs. multiple) and by specific cognitive domain (attention and working memory, executive functions, language, memory, and visuospatial skills). Indeed, PD MCI is a highly heterogeneous condition, notwithstanding the fact that increased age, motor disease severity, non-tremor-dominant phenotype, and lower educational levels all seem to be robustly associated with MCI risk. Whether PD MCI inevitably deteriorates to a state of dementia is still an unanswered question. Evidence suggests that individual cognitive subtypes have

BOX 3.1 **Movement Disorders Society Task Force Criteria for Mild Cognitive Impairment in Parkinson's Disease**

Inclusion Criteria

PD diagnosis based on UKPDS brain bank criteria

- Gradual decline in cognitive ability reported by patient or informant or observed by clinician
- Cognitive deficits demonstrable on neuropsychological testing or a global cognitive scale
- Cognitive impairment does not interfere significantly with functional ability

Level I criteria: Abbreviated assessment

- Impairment on global cognitive scale validated in PD (e.g., MoCA) or impairment on at least two tests from a limited neuropsychological battery (two or more tests per domain or five or more domains tested)

Level 2 criteria: Comprehensive assessment

- Neuropsychological testing includes two tests within each of five cognitive domains (attention and working memory, executive functions, language, memory, visuospatial skills)
- Impairment on at least two tests: either two impaired tests within one domain or one test in two different domains
- Impairment demonstrated by: a score 1 or 2 standard deviation below appropriate norms, or significant decline on serial cognitive testing, or significant decline from estimated premorbid levels

Subtype classification for PD MCI: Comprehensive assessment required

- Single domain: Abnormalities on two tests within a single cognitive domain
- Multiple domain: Abnormalities on at least one test in two or more domains

Exclusion Criteria

Diagnosis of PD dementia based on Movement Disorders Society dementia criteria

Another explanation for cognitive impairment (e.g., delirium, depression, medication side effects)

Other PD-related factors that have a significant impact on cognitive testing (e.g., motor impairment, anxiety, sleepiness, psychosis)

MCI, mild cognitive impairment; MoCA, Montreal Cognitive Assessment; PD, Parkinson's disease; UKPDS, United Kingdom Parkinson's Disease Society.

Source: Reprinted with permission from Goldman JG, Williams-Gray C, Barker RA, Duda JE, Galvin JE. The spectrum of cognitive impairment in Lewy body disease. *Mov Disord* 2014;29(5):608–621.

differing prognoses, with executive deficits alone not clearly associated with dementia, whereas posterior, cortically based deficits (i.e., memory and visuospatial dysfunctions) possibly represent the early stages of a dementing process. Thus, such patients should be referred for formal cognitive testing in order to specify the number and type of affected domains because the results may be helpful in prognostication.

MANAGEMENT

The key to management is identification of the problem and then education of the patient and family. Pharmacological strategies may not be suitable for all patients. This relates to tolerability issues and side effects, lack of benefit, and costs. Where appropriate, pharmacologic treatment of PD patients with cognitive impairment is aimed at improving cognition and controlling the associated behavioral disturbances.

For cognitive deficits, all the marketed cholinesterase inhibitors (e.g., donepezil, rivastigmine, and galantamine) have been tested in people with PD who have mild to moderate dementia. The strongest evidence is for rivastigmine (Table 3.1). Due to the risk of cardiac dysrhythmia, an ECG is suggested prior to starting treatment.

Memantine is an N-methyl-D-aspartate receptor antagonist (Table 3.1) approved for the treatment of Alzheimer's disease, which showed modest efficacy in patients with PD and dementia. Treating MCI has been less well studied, although several trials are ongoing.

TABLE 3.1 **Medications for Management of Patients with PD and Cognitive Impairment**

Medication	Daily Dose (mg)
To enhance cognitive abilities	
Donepezil	5–10
Rivastigmine	9–12
Galantamine	8–16
Memantine	10–20
To control psychotic symptoms	
Quetiapine	12.5–300
Clozapine	6.25–75

Drugs for cognitive impairment may also have a benefit on behavioral disturbances. Cholinesterase inhibitors can reduce hallucinations, often very effectively, but they will not reduce psychosis. In some individuals, hallucinations and delusions may be severe enough to require treatment with atypical antipsychotics, such as quetiapine and clozapine (all are off-label use) (Table 3.1). Quetiapine is usually tried as first-line treatment for its ease of use and relative lack of side effects. However, evidence suggests that the most effective results on PD psychosis are obtained with clozapine (although use of this drug can be inconvenient due to the requirement for regular blood monitoring because of the risk of agranulocytosis with this drug).

With regard to mood issues, although there is evidence that tricyclics, such as amitriptyline and nortriptyline, may have greater benefit, they should be avoided in PD patients with cognitive impairment because of their anticholinergic effects and hence the potential to worsen cognition. Thus, selective serotonin reuptake inhibitors or serotonin norepinephrine reuptake inhibitors are commonly preferred. To date, there is no good evidence for superiority of one antidepressant over another in PD.

PRACTICAL ISSUES

People with cognitive impairment as a complication of their PD have increased vulnerability in several respects and can be open to manipulation, coercion, or may themselves act against their own best interests. On the other hand, there are situations in which there is a need to protect others from patients' choices and behavior. Except in cases in which statutory obligation exists, clinicians must use their judgment as to when functional capacity is best assessed, particularly with respect to driving capacity, which can be an emotive issue. A diagnosis of PD does not prevent the patient from driving; however, the presence of cognitive impairment may significantly affect driving safety. A decision about driving fitness in PD should be a joint process including the neurologist, the neuropsychologist, the patient, and caregivers. It is advisable to talk with patients and families at an early stage about all these issues, and future planning about important decisions, such as making a provision for enduring power of attorney, is best done well ahead of time.

- Cognitive impairment and dementia are common during the course of PD.
- Behavioral disturbances, mood change, and psychotic symptoms often herald or accompany cognitive decline in PD.
- Therapeutic strategies include administration of cholinesterase inhibitors to improve cognitive function and antidepressants/atypical antipsychotics to control behavioral disturbance.
- Conversations with patients and families about ethical issues, increased vulnerability, and how decisions will be made in the future should be done sooner rather than later.

Further Reading

Aarsland D, Taylor JP, Weintraub D. Psychiatric issues in cognitive impairment. *Mov Disord* 2014;29(5):651–662.

Emre M, Ford PJ, Bilgiç B, Uç EY. Cognitive impairment and dementia in Parkinson's disease: Practical issues and management. *Mov Disord* 2014;29(5):663–672.

Goldman JG, Williams-Gray C, Barker RA, Duda JE, Galvin JE. The spectrum of cognitive impairment in Lewy body disease. *Mov Disord* 2014;29(5):608–621.

Marras C, Tröster AI, Kulisevsky J, Stebbins GT. The tools of the trade: A state of the art "How to Assess Cognition" in the patient with Parkinson's disease. *Mov Disord* 2014;29(5):584–596.

4   Beyond Tremor, Slowness, and Stiffness

Robertus M. A. de Bie

The patient is a 74-year-old woman who has had Parkinson's disease for the past 6 years. Before the motor symptoms started, she had pain in her limbs, especially the left leg. The severity of the pain fluctuates. She may experience several hours of severe pain alternating with periods of less pain. She describes the pain as fierce and stabbing. The patient denies a temporal relationship between the time of medication intake and the severity of the pain. She is unable to sleep, although this is not always due to pain. She falls asleep easily in the day. Her past medical history included surgery for a carpal tunnel syndrome on the left side and gout. She uses levodopa/carbidopa/entacapone 150/37.5/200 mg TID, ropinirole sustained release 8 mg daily, levodopa/carbidopa sustained release 100/25 mg daily at bedtime, and allopurinol. The physical examination did not demonstrate signs of a local cause of the pain, such as inflammation, radicular syndrome, or a polyneuropathy.

What do you do now?

NONMOTOR SYMPTOMS IN PARKINSON'S DISEASE

The motor symptoms of Parkinson's disease (PD) are characterized by the progression of tremor, rigidity, bradykinesia, and postural disturbances. The disease may be accompanied by a variety of nonmotor symptoms, such as autonomic, cognitive, psychiatric, sensory, and sleep disorders. These may even precede the motor symptoms, and in a considerable proportion of patients nonmotor symptoms are the major determinant of disability, especially in the more advanced stages of the disease. This patient is experiencing two nonmotor symptoms—pain and insomnia.

Pain in PD can be discerned according to the following descriptive categories: musculoskeletal pain, pain and discomfort localized to the territory of a nerve or nerve root, pain as part of dystonia, pain of presumed central origin, and discomfort accompanying akathisia. The first task is to decide whether the pain is related to PD or represents an unrelated but important medical condition requiring further evaluation. Pain related to PD may occur as a wearing-off phenomenon, as a beginning-of-dose or end-of-dose phenomenon, or as a peak-dose effect of dopaminergic medication. If a temporal relationship between pain and the medication schedule is recognized, the emphasis should be on adjusting dopaminergic medication accordingly.

Insomnia is very common in PD, and the most frequent cause is untreated or undertreated nocturnal parkinsonism. Other causes may be mentally activating drugs (e.g., selegiline), stimulant drugs (e.g., methylphenidate), and alcohol and coffee consumption. Nocturnal parkinsonism is very responsive to levodopa therapy. Nighttime insomnia may cause excessive daytime sleepiness, but levodopa and dopamine agonists may also be considered as possible sources. PD patients frequently act out their dreams while asleep, which indicates rapid eye movement (REM) sleep behavior disorder. This may precede the other symptoms by many years. In general, if the patient awakens feeling tired after a night's sleep, REM sleep behavior disorder is not an adequate explanation. Treat the disorder if the activity presents a potential danger to the patient or the partner. Bedtime clonazepam 0.25–0.5 mg is an effective treatment for REM sleep behavior disorder. It is important to discern REM sleep behavior disorder from nocturnal hallucinations and nocturnal confusion because the treatments are markedly different.

In this case, we asked the patient to register the severity of pain (0 = no pain and 10 = most severe pain) every 30 minutes for 7 days. Subsequently, we calculated the mean score per 30 minutes (i.e., from 7 to 7:30 a.m., from 7:30 to 8 a.m., and so forth). We made a graph of the scores, which demonstrated clearly, also to the patient, the relation between the time of medication intake and the

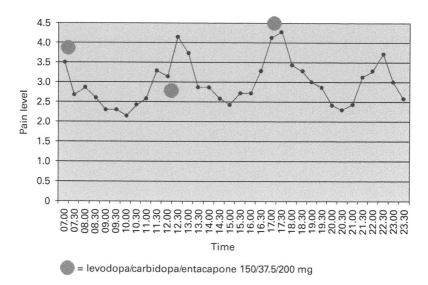

FIGURE 4.1 Graph of pain level during the day (mean of 7 days; 0 – no pain and 10 = most severe pain).

level of pain (Fig. 4.1). We increased the administration of levodopa/carbidopa/entacapone from three times per day to four times per day.

OTHER NONMOTOR SYMPTOMS

Depression

Prevalence estimates for depression vary widely, typically between 20% and 40%, due to differences in study populations, definitions, and criteria for symptom attribution. Assessing depression in PD is challenging, partially due to the overlap between depression and the PD symptoms. In this context, nonsomatic symptoms of depression discriminate best between depressed and nondepressed patients. Only scarce data are available regarding the choices for an antidepressant in PD. In a small study, nortriptyline was shown to be efficacious. Selective serotonin reuptake inhibitors may be less effective in PD than in the general elderly population, but they are often used to treat depression in PD. Venlafaxine is considered to be efficacious. Also, the dopamine agonist pramipexole was shown to be efficacious for the treatment of depressive symptoms in PD.

Autonomic Dysfunction

The definition of orthostatic hypotension is made by consensus and is a fall of 20 mmHg systolic or 10 mmHg diastolic blood pressures within 3 minutes of active standing or head up tilt. The prevalence in PD is approximately 30%. Although many different treatments for orthostatic hypotension have been investigated, controlled trials are sparse and are generally conducted on small sample sizes. Therefore, the mainstay of management is nonpharmacological and consists of the advice to avoid orthostatic hypotension and instructions on physical countermaneuvers for maintaining adequate blood pressure during orthostasis. If these fail, fludrocortisone or midodrine may be prescribed.

For urinary symptoms, increased frequency, urgency, and urge incontinence, along with nocturia and bladder retention, are frequent in the advanced stages of the disease. Advise the patient to avoid large intakes of water or natural diuretics such as coffee before bedtime. Peripherally acting anticholinergic drugs (e.g., oxybutynin), antispasmodic agents, and alpha-1 agonists can be used for urinary urgency, although these drugs have not been specifically evaluated in PD.

Constipation is extremely common in PD, and managing it is important to ensure adequate absorption of levodopa. Management includes adequate fluid intake, exercise, diet, and stool softeners. Laxatives and enemas may be required.

Drooling

Patients may suffer from sialorrhea due to dysphagia (i.e., an inability to swallow saliva normally). Simple remedies include chewing gum. Oral glycopyrrolate 1 mg TID is an effective and safe therapy for sialorrhea in PD. Another effective treatment is intraglandular botulinum toxin injections performed by an experienced physician; however, care must be taken not to exacerbate dysphagia. In exceptional cases of extreme sialorrhea, consider radiotherapy of the glands.

Fatigue

Patients with PD have greater physical and mental fatigue. Although fatigue may be a consequence of the motor symptoms or secondary to other nonmotor symptoms such as depression, anxiety, excessive daytime sleepiness, or apathy, it may be a primary symptom, independent of these other comorbidities. Levodopa and dopamine agonists may induce excessive daytime sleepiness. Although the phenomenon is poorly understood, fatigue may be very disabling. Two small controlled trials have shown that nortriptyline and methylphenidate may improve fatigue in PD.

- Always ask about these nonmotor symptoms.
- If present, determine if they fluctuate; many are worse in the "off" period.
- The most common cause for insomnia is untreated or undertreated nocturnal parkinsonism, which is very responsive to levodopa therapy.
- If a medical condition requiring further evaluation is excluded and a temporal relationship between pain and the medication schedule is recognized, the emphasis should be on adjusting dopaminergic medication accordingly.

Further Reading

Ahlskog JE. *Parkinson's Disease Treatment Guide for Physicians*. New York, NY: Oxford University Press, 2009.

Seppi K, Weintraub D, Coelho M, et al. The Movement Disorder Society evidence-based medicine review update: Treatments for the non-motor symptoms of Parkinson's disease. *Mov Disord* 2011;26(Suppl 3):S42–S80.

5 Is Now the Time ... ?

Robertus M. A. de Bie

A 68-year-old man who has had Parkinson's disease for 8 years recently heard about deep brain stimulation and wants to know whether he could benefit. He has medication-induced motor response fluctuations. If the medication kicks in, the patient is independent and even helps his son on their farm, but when he is off medication, he needs help dressing. There are no problems with postural stability, no freezing of gait, and no complaints regarding cognitive performance. With a higher dose of ropinirole—a dopamine agonist—he suffered from uncontrollable gambling, and subsequently this was stopped. He now takes levodopa/carbidopa 100/25 mg 1.5 tablets seven times per day, each time together with entacapone 200 mg. At approximately 11 p.m., he takes levodopa/carbidopa 200/50 mg in a controlled-release formulation, and sometimes he takes 2 tablets of Madopar Dispersible 100/25 mg during the night. He uses amantadine 100 mg TID because of dyskinesias, which are reduced but still bothersome.

What do you do now?

WHOM TO REFER FOR SURGERY

The first experience with Parkinson's disease (PD) patients treated with continuous deep brain stimulation (DBS) of the subthalamic nucleus (STN) was published in 1995. Since then, thousands of PD patients have been treated with DBS. Randomized controlled trials have shown (1) the superior efficacy of STN DBS compared to best medical treatment, (2) the superiority of STN DBS over unilateral pallidotomy, and (3) that thalamic DBS is more efficacious than thalamotomy. However, pallidotomy and thalamotomy may still be considered in a select group of patients (e.g., if DBS is not possible).

Three DBS targets are used for PD, and all three are part of the cortex–basal ganglia–thalamus–cortex system. DBS of the STN and DBS of the internal segment of the globus pallidus (GPI) are used to reduce parkinsonism (hypokinesia, rigidity, and tremor), dystonia, PD pain, and PD-medication–induced involuntary movements (dyskinesia). Differences on cognitive function and mood as side-effects may occur in visuomotor speed and depression. Average PD medication can be decreased more after STN DBS compared to GPI DBS (32% vs. 18%). In addition, stimulation amplitudes and pulse widths are lower for STN than for GPI DBS, allowing for longer intervals between pulse-generator replacements with STN DBS.

DBS of the ventral intermediate nucleus (VIM)/thalamus is used to improve tremor. The efficacy of VIM/thalamic DBS for the treatment of tremor was never compared prospectively with STN or GPI DBS. However, it seems wise to choose the STN DBS in cases of tremor, especially in young patients, because eventually they will suffer from other motor symptoms.

Currently, most physicians choose the STN as the DBS target for PD patients. However, there may be reasons to deviate from the standard target. In advanced PD, for example, it is worthwhile to consider GPI DBS if STN DBS is not an option. Also, in an elderly patient with medication-resistant tremor-dominant PD and (mild) cognitive impairments, one may consider VIM/thalamic DBS.

DBS does not help for all PD symptoms. PD affects the motor, autonomic, cognitive, affective, and sensory systems. The motor symptoms are characterized by the progression of tremor, rigidity, bradykinesia, and postural disturbances. These symptoms form the hallmark of PD. However, currently it is clear that nonmotor symptoms are the major determinant of disability in the advanced stages of the disease. As outlined previously, DBS improves specific PD symptoms—that is, not all symptoms. The clinical picture of PD is very heterogeneous among patients, and when considering DBS treatment, it is crucial to determine which symptoms cause (major) disability. When evaluating a patient for DBS surgery, consider that there may be incapacitating symptoms that may arise within the not-too-distant future (Fig. 5.1). Portents are, for example, falls, hallucinations, and impaired attention.

Over time, new PD symptoms emerge. These may be more disabling than the (initial) motor symptoms. Treatment becomes more complex when the disease progresses. Criteria for consideration of DBS treatment are as follows:

- Idiopathic PD, instead of multiple system atrophy or progressive supranuclear palsy
- Levodopa-responsive motor symptoms (hypo/bradykinesia, tremor, dystonia, and pain)
- Drug-resistant tremor
- Not for balance or speech problems only
- Hoehn and Yahr stage less than 5 during the best "on" medication phase
- (Threatening) impaired functional health
- Benefit of adjusting drug treatments unlikely
- No cognitive problems
- No depression or psychosis
- No contraindications for (functional neuro-)surgery

The patient mentioned previously seems to qualify for DBS. When evaluating a patient for DBS, most teams do at least the following examinations:

1. First is a standardized assessment of PD motor symptoms; mostly this is a so-called "off/on" medication phase assessment. The "off" medication

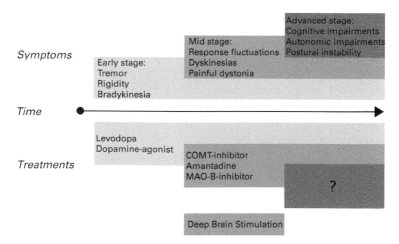

FIGURE 5.1 Stages of Parkinson's disease. Three stages can be distinguished: early, mid, and advanced. The pathophysiological mechanisms that underlie the symptoms are different for each stage, and such treatments are different according to the stage of the disease. COMT, catechol-*O*-methyltransferase; MAO-B, monoamine oxidase B.

phase is defined as the condition of the patient after withholding PD medication for 12 hours (overnight) and being awake for at least 1 hour. The "on" medication phase is the condition 1 hour after a levodopa dose. This dose should bring about an "on" phase, and typically a suprathreshold levodopa dose is used. This amount of levodopa is based on the patient's usual first morning dose. In the standardized "off" and "on" phases, scores on the Unified Parkinson's Disease Rating Scale (UPDRS-III) and a dyskinesia rating scale are recorded. Response to levodopa is universally accepted as the single best outcome predictor for response to DBS.

2. Brain imaging is done, such as a computed tomography or magnetic resonance imaging scan.

3. Blood analysis for prothrombin time, activated partial thromboplastin time, and a complete blood count are obtained.

4. Neuropsychological testing is done, although there is no consensus regarding the choice of tests and the level of severity of cognitive impairments that would exclude patients from receiving DBS. However, it seems wise not to operate on clearly cognitively affected patients.

It is very important to extensively inform the patient and family regarding the surgical procedures because the patient is awake during surgery and good patient cooperation improves the results of surgery. Having a burr hole drilled in one's skull while awake is quite a surreal experience. It is also essential to prepare the patient and family for the course of events in the months following surgery (i.e., adjusting medication schedule and DBS settings) and to anticipate unrealistic expectations.

In many centers, neurologists take part in the surgery. They perform the intraoperative physiological localization of the DBS target and the clinical testing. The person who performs this task should be able to do the following:

· Interpret microelectrode recordings (if these are used)
· Accurately assess PD symptoms and signs, including dystonia
· Recognize the side effects of medication
· (Immediately) recognize signs of complications and side effects of stimulation
· Know the functional anatomy of the brain area in question

For the clinical assessment during surgery, rigidity, bradykinesia, and tremor are used; therefore, a patient should be in the "off" phase. For maximal reproducibility of PD signs and effects of electrical stimulation, the signs should be assessed during surgery in the same manner (same tests and same activation maneuvers) and by one examiner. The patient's clinical condition may change during surgery due to fatigue and less motivation.

The rates of surgical complications are quite variable in the literature. The experience of the surgical team is a key factor in reducing the risk of surgical complications. The most frequent procedure-related adverse effects were mental status and behavioral changes (almost 20% following STN DBS, including transient effects), followed by infection (2.0%) and symptomatic intracranial hemorrhage (2.0%). Examples of DBS hardware problems are lead erosion (without infection), lead fracture, and lead migration. Permanent stimulation-related adverse effects—also possibly disease-related—are dysarthria (almost 13%), apraxia of eyelid opening (10%), and cognitive decline (6%). The postoperative management can be very complex, for example, due to a nonmotor dopamine withdrawal syndrome and impulse-control disorders.

KEY POINTS TO REMEMBER

- DBS improves not all but only specific PD symptoms, especially bradykinesia, tremor, dystonia, and pain.
- Medication-resistant tremor can improve with DBS.
- Response to levodopa is universally accepted as the single best outcome predictor for response to DBS.
- The most frequent procedure-related adverse effects are mental status and behavioral changes.

Further Reading

Bain P, Aziz T, Liu X, Nandi D. *Deep Brain Stimulation*. New York, NY: Oxford University Press, 2009.

Thevathasan W, Gregory R. Deep brain stimulation for movement disorders. *Practical Neurol* 2010;10:16–26.

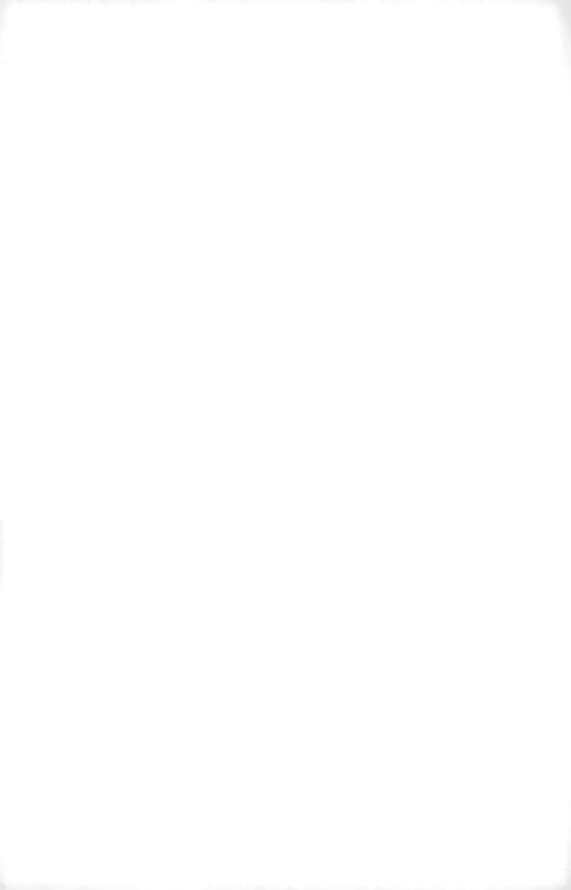

6 When Less Is More

Richard A. Walsh

You meet a 78-year-old male patient with long-standing Parkinson's disease for a routine review. He was diagnosed 20 years ago and enjoyed many years of good motor function, enabling him to continue working to retirement and remain independent until 2 years ago. At that point, evolving cognitive impairment and loss of postural reflexes required the placement of a carer to help his wife with his activities of daily living.

He will still get a good "on" response to levodopa, lasting between 2 and 3 hours, although often contaminated by bothersome generalized dyskinesia. Amantadine did reduce this some years ago, and he continues on 100 mg TDS. He can fall due to freezing in the "on" or "off" condition. Hallucinations have become increasingly common, with increasingly limited insight. His wife mentions significant social embarrassment due to increasing dysarthria and drooling for which she will bring a number of hand towels in her handbag, along with a spare shirt. Sleep disruption is increasingly common, often waking his wife.

What do you do now?

PALLIATION IN PARKINSON'S DISEASE

Palliative Neurology as a Subspecialty

For the layperson, palliative care is strongly associated with a diagnosis of "terminal" cancer or the end stages of some other terminal illness. This association is generally the result of experiences with other family members. It is therefore important, when dealing with patients with neurodegenerative disorders, to have a discussion at an early stage about the different role of the palliative care team in neurological disease. Specifically, it should be emphasized that consultation with a colleague with an interest in palliative neurology is not a precursor of imminent rapid decline or death. The role of palliative care in neurological disease represents an acceptance of our current limitations with respect to preserving function and the importance of sustaining comfort and quality of life. In most countries, palliative care remains a general specialty, although palliative neurology and related publications have demonstrated recent traction as a subspecialty of importance. This is a positive trend that will become increasingly important as the prevalence of neurodegenerative disease increases with our aging populations.

When Palliation Becomes Relevant in Parkinson's Disease

The management of Parkinson's disease (PD) in its early and middle stages is different from that of atypical parkinsonian conditions in one critical respect. In PD, levodopa and other dopaminergic therapies offer the potential of a good symptomatic response in most patients, often providing many years, or even decades, of effective symptom control. Unfortunately, this is not the case for related disorders such as multiple system atrophy (MSA) or progressive supranuclear palsy (PSP), in which there is an emphasis on maximizing comfort in the face of progressive disability from the beginning, although a small group of patients will experience a transient improvement with levodopa. In these related disorders, early institution of a palliative approach is important. In the later stages of PD, in which symptoms nonresponsive to levodopa become more prominent, a palliative care approach is equally beneficial.

Rationalization of Drug Therapies

Despite the availability of effective pharmacological therapies and deep-brain stimulation in PD, there is a point for most patients at which the addition of more drugs or increasing doses is of no value. In fact, once this point is reached, greater pharmacotherapy can be detrimental, such as causing increasing somnolence, triggering new hallucinations, or exacerbating orthostatic hypotension. In the first decade of treating PD, the natural course is to add layer upon layer of treatment as the disease evolves, often with a dopamine agonist and perhaps adding a monoamine oxidase B (MAO-B) inhibitor, then levodopa, and perhaps amantadine later. With advancing age and the almost inevitable emergence of cognitive impairment, the law of diminishing marginal returns will determine that further efforts to claw back hours of effective "on" time are often frustrated by tolerability issues or worsening dyskinesia without a meaningful improvement in quality of life. It is at this stage, which may become apparent over a number of visits, that a peeling away process is of greater value. The progressive elimination of less useful and more toxic drugs is often the first palliative step that a neurologist treating PD will take (Table 6.1).

TABLE 6.1 **Palliative Measures to Consider in Advanced Parkinson's Disease**[a]

Symptom	Intervention
Siallorrhea	Ipratropium inhaler sprayed under the tongue. Botulinum toxin to parotid and submandibular glands can be effective but can be uncomfortable and response variable, particularly in the absence of ultrasound guidance.
Confusion, agitation, progression of cognitive impairment	Wean or reduce anticholinergics, amantadine, selegiline, and dopamine agonists in that order as appropriate.
Depression and anxiety	Use SSRIs and SNRIs over tricyclic antidepressants, which are more likely to be associated with confusion.
REM sleep behavior disorder (RBD) and fragmented sleep patterns	Clonazepam 0.5–2 mg nocte can be very effective in reducing RBD and also helpful as a general night sedative.
Falls	Where frequent, encourage the use of a wheelchair for longer distances and to facilitate care and options outside the home.
Troublesome hallucinations	If drug reduction as for confusion, agitation, and progression of cognitive impairment is ineffective, use quetiapine or clozapine in preference to other neuroleptics; typically effective in low doses.
Somnolence	Drug withdrawal is again the mainstay. Most commonly associated with dopamine agonists but also seen at peak of levodopa cycle. Encourage judicious use of "catnaps" during the day.

(continued)

TABLE 6.1 **Continued**

Symptom	Intervention
Urinary urge and frequency	In men, coexistent prostatism is common and urinary symptoms will often improve with use of an alpha-blocker such as tamsulosin. Anticholinergics can exacerbate cognitive impairment; newer agents such as mirabegron, a B_3 adrenoceptor agonist, can be considered.
Pain	Pain perception from any source can be magnified in a low dopamine state. If "off" period pain, manipulation of dopaminergic therapies may help if room to maneuver. No specific analgesics are otherwise recommended, although special caution with regard to constipation and opiates is required.
Fatigue	Hugely troublesome symptom without a ready solution. More pervasive than episodic somnolence and not always associated with a desire to sleep. Likely a multifactorial phenomenon in this population. Encourage good sleep hygiene, eliminate depression as a factor, and ensure it is not an "off" phenomenon that may respond to dopaminergic medication.
Dysphagia	Common and generally managed by dietary modification and compensatory strategies. Although aspiration pneumonia is a common cause of death, placement of PEG tube is rarely required or appropriate.

[a]Any of these disease features can be seen alone or in combination in patients with otherwise uncomplicated Parkinson's disease, but as a group of disease features, they are most commonly seen in patients with advanced disease in whom a palliative approach is appropriate.

PEG, percutaneous endoscopic gastrostomy; SNRIs, serotonin norepinephrine reuptake inhibitors; SSRIs, selective serotonin reuptake inhibitors.

The order in which drugs are withdrawn should begin with the agent tolerated the poorest in the aging brain. Despite any potential anxiety to remove any drug immediately in a hallucinating patient, a slow wean over weeks is preferable to avoid precipitation of a withdrawal worsening or paradoxical confusion that can be unpredictable. Anticholinergics are particularly troublesome in older patients with PD, contributing to worsening amnestic features, confusion, and hallucinations. Many neurologists avoid anticholinergics in patients older than age 65 years, although occasionally some patients in their mid-seventies with relatively preserved cognition will continue to obtain a very useful tremor response with a drug in this class.

Amantadine is another drug that one should have a low threshold for discontinuing in a patient with troublesome hallucinations. Rebound worsening of dyskinesia can occur, placing the treating physician in a difficult situation. The lesser of two evils can be lowering total daily levodopa dose with a tolerance of greater bradykinesia over hallucinations.

In a vulnerable brain, the MAO-B inhibitor selegiline, with its amphetamine breakdown products, can contribute to sleep disturbance and hallucinations. In a patient with more than 15 years of disease, its contribution to overall motor function is very small, and it should be discontinued if necessary.

Consideration for the Carer

The definition of palliation reflects the importance of maximizing quality of life for both the patient and the carer. The significant carer burden is well described in PD, characterized by increased stress, fatigue, and even mortality. Unlike in conditions such as motor neuron disease and incurable cancers, in which communication and cognition are often relatively preserved to the end, carers living with people in the advanced stages of PD must cope with a complex and multifaceted illness. More than 60% of patients with PD of more than 15 years' duration will have dementia, and this increases to more than 80% at 20 years. Full dependence from a motor and cognitive perspective along with an absence of feedback or meaningful communication place an extra burden on this carer group.

To this situation can be added the common disruption of sleep patterns, florid hallucinations, incontinence, and a drug regimen that can be extremely sensitive to time and diet. It can be understood why caregiver burnout is a common but often unrecognized phenomenon among PD carers, who are themselves generally elderly and dealing with their own medical issues. The effects of this phenomenon can be mitigated very effectively by the use of regular respite admissions to local care facilities, providing a chance to rest in addition to a change of scene for a patient who is often housebound. Studies examining the prevalence of caregiver morbidity in PD have shown that access to community services, including respite care, is poor and, where available, uptake among carers can be poor. Reluctance to accept assistance can be due to pride, reluctance to relinquish care, a fear of losing privacy, or a feeling of guilt. Linking carers with a carer network, where available, can be useful in this regard, allowing carers to share the psychological burden but also learn coping strategies from others in a similar situation.

In neurodegenerative diseases, there are many years during which carer burnout can become a significant problem. In more rapidly progressive conditions, such as MSA and PSP, there is less time for this to occur, but the intensity of the care required is greater. The central position of a carer in the management of these conditions means that the neglect of the carer's needs serves to diminish both the quality of life of the carer and that of the patient. There are a number of ways in which carers can be supported in their role:

In This Case

Although the man in this case has a large amount of "off" time daily, any effort to reduce this is going to be beset with challenges. There is a need to wean amantadine due to cognitive impairment; a reduction of 100 mg every week is reasonable. This will worsen dyskinesia, a factor only exacerbated by any effort to increase "on" time with more levodopa. Furthermore, one would have to ask what improvement in quality of life would be obtained; falls are frequent even in the best "on" condition, so nothing will be achieved in attempting to maximize "on" time. Night disruption could be improved with a small dose of clonazepam, reducing REM sleep behavior disorder and facilitating longer periods of sleep. Caution is required when prescribing clonazepam; failure to wake can result in enuresis and more sheets for the carer to change, and attempts to mobilize at night through sedation can increase the risk of a fall and injury. Botulinum toxin may improve the troublesome drooling. A discussion with both patient and carer about expectations, reasonable aims of therapy, and planning for the future is required.

KEY POINTS TO REMEMBER

- A palliative phase exists in PD, lasting on average 2 or 3 years, in which drug-responsive features wane and cognitive impairment becomes increasingly prominent.
- The natural history of PD produces a predominance of nonmotor complications in the later years that can often be more disabling than the motor complications due to their impact on quality of life. These features are frustratingly challenging to manage but must not be ignored as a result.
- When dementia and hallucinations become established and bothersome, a slow wean of any drugs that may be contributing should be undertaken, starting with anticholinergics and amantadine.

- Introduce the discussion about planning for enduring power of attorney at an early stage to avoid more complicated, expensive, and lengthy proceedings later when capacity is lost.
- Recognition of the carer burden is an important facet of the palliative neurology consultation, which should target resources to limit carer burnout in recognition of the critical role of the carer.

Further Reading

Hasson F, Kernohan WG, McLaughlin M, et al. An exploration into the palliative and end-of-life experiences of carers of people with Parkinson's disease. *Palliat Med* 2010;24(7):731–736.

Hely MA, Reid WGJ, Adena MA, Halliday GM, Morris JGL. The Sydney multicenter study of Parkinson's disease: The inevitability of dementia at 20 years. *Mov Disord* 2008;23:837–844.

Miyasaki JM, Kluger B. Palliative care for Parkinson's disease: Has the time come? *Curr Neurol Neurosci Rep* 2015;15(5):26.

Richfield EW, Jones EJ, Alty JE. Palliative care for Parkinson's disease: A summary of the evidence and future directions. *Palliat Med* 2013 Oct;27(9):805–810.

7 "Are My Children at Risk, Doctor?"

Richard A. Walsh

You are reviewing an unmarried 42-year-old woman with a 3-year history of left foot cramping with prolonged exercise. This problem has been increasingly bothersome. Over time, she has become aware of diminishing dexterity in her left hand with intermittent tremor at rest. She has little upper limb disability, being right-handed, although she is conscious of the tremor, which can be socially embarrassing. She has no cognitive concerns. On further questioning, she tells you that her father had Parkinson's disease, but he was only affected in his 70s. She has six siblings, none of whom are similarly affected.

On examination, she has good facial expression. She has very mild but definite bradykinesia for all hand movements on the left, with rigidity present only with coactivation. She walks well with evidence of dystonic posturing after 10 lengths of the corridor outside your examination room. Reflexes are brisk throughout. You discuss Parkinson's disease. She asks about genetic testing in the family.

What do you do now?

GENETIC TESTING IN PARKINSON'S DISEASE

As many as 10% of patients with Parkinson's disease (PD) will report a positive family history. Despite the existence of a well-recognized and established group of uncommon dominantly and recessively inherited genes associated with monogenic PD, it is far more likely that patients with such a positive family history will not be found to carry one of these. There has also been little success in expanding this group of inherited genes associated with monogenic parkinsonism to account for the large group in whom no gene can be identified. It is possible that a number of genetic susceptibilities or risk factors may appear in an individual, and such complexity may be important in making the genetic underpinnings of apparently familial PD elusive. Such genetic susceptibility factors, including polymorphisms in the *SNCA* and *LRRK2* genes, have been identified in large genome-wide association studies of large PD populations compared with control groups, although the individual odds ratio for each is low. The relative contribution of additional genetic factors, the number required to manifest disease, and the additive or protective role of environmental factors remain unclear. Carriers of single mutations in the glucocerebrosidase gene (*GBA*), associated with Gaucher's disease in the homozygous state, have a fivefold risk of developing PD. Unlike the monogenic forms of PD shown in Table 7.1, it is unclear if this finding represents a genetic susceptibility factor or a poorly penetrant form of monogenic PD. An important factor in the effort to establish genetic factors in familial PD is the likely genetic and pathological heterogeneity, with a number of separate disease processes giving rise to a similar end-phenotype, making it difficult to establish a group to study with homogeneous genetics and pathophysiology.

WHAT DOES THIS MEAN FOR THE PATIENT?

From a practical perspective, for a given patient sitting in front of you, the identification of a specific genetic cause has no implications for management. Treatment with either medical or surgical approaches is not influenced to any significant degree, with the same principles being followed in patients with and without a monogenic cause of their disease. As with any genetic testing, however, there is some value in pursuing underlying genetic studies to assist with prognostication (discussed later) and to provide counseling to other family members and couples considering conception. Of greater importance, perhaps, is the role of genetic testing in the advancement of our knowledge about the pathophysiology of PD and the search for disease-modifying therapies. Although of no direct value to the patient with whom you are talking, many patients will consent to testing on a research basis if it may benefit similarly affected patients in the future.

TABLE 7.1   Monogenic Forms of Parkinson's Disease Presenting with a Largely Typical Parkinsonian Phenotype

Gene [Locus] (Protein)	Inheritance	Presentation
LRRK2 [PARK8] (Lrrk2 or dardarin)	AD	High prevalence in North African and Ashkenazi Jewish populations. Phenotype largely indistinguishable from idiopathic PD with late onset. Lower incidence of dementia and abduction–adduction leg tremor reported.
SNCA [PARK1/4] (alpha-synuclein)	AD	Prominent cognitive impairment/ dementia, myoclonus, and dysautonomia. Faster progression than in sporadic PD.
VPS35 (vacuolar protein sorting 35 homolog)	AD	Typical phenotype, although with earlier age of onset. Dementia is uncommon in reported cases.
PRKN [PARK2] (Parkin)	AR	Onset typically before age 45 years; lower limb dystonia; very good levodopa response with prominent motor fluctuations. Relatively preserved cognition. Heterozygous state also linked to PD, although causal link not established.
PINK1 [PARK6] (PTEN-induced kinase 1)	AR	Early onset, prominent dystonia, pyramidal signs in some with good sleep benefit
DJ-1 [PARK7] (Daisuke–Junko-1)	AR	Early-onset with good levodopa response and relatively preserved cognition with neuropsychiatric features.

AD, autosomal dominant; LRRK, leucine-rich repeat kinase 2; PD, Parkinson's disease; VPS35, vacuolar protein sorting 35.

MONOGENIC PARKINSON'S DISEASE

Genes Associated with Autosomal Dominant Inheritance

SNCA (PARK1/2)

This was the first gene confirmed to be associated with monogenic PD after its identification in Greek and Italian families approximately 20 years ago, and it now represents the second most common cause of dominant inheritance after *LRRK2* mutations. Duplications, triplications, and a small number of identified point mutations have been described in association with early onset PD. The phenotype is characterized by prominent cortical involvement with myoclonus and dementia present at an earlier stage than would be expected in typical sporadic PD. Prominent dysautonomia is another reported feature, along with a tendency to exhibit diminishing levodopa response over time.

Leucine-Rich Repeat Kinase 2 (*LRRK2, PARK8*)

This is the most common cause of autosomal dominant PD. First discovered in 2004, *LRRK2* mutations account for greater than 5% of familial PD and are also found in up to 3% of apparently sporadic cases with variations among different populations studied. Prevalence is higher in northern African Arabic and Jewish kindreds, in which *LRRK2* mutations may account for as many as 40% of familial cases. The clinical picture can be identical to that seen in sporadic PD. Penetrance in carriers increases by approximately 10% with each passing decade in adult life, increasing to greater than 70% by 80 years of age, although penetrance data may differ between the pathogenic point mutations described to date.

VPS35

Mutations in this gene are a recently described cause of monogenic PD that is likely to represent less than 1% of familial cases. Unlike the *SNCA* and *LRRK2* genes, *VPS35* mutations were identified using next-generation sequencing techniques in whole exome sequencing of Australian and Swiss pedigrees. The phenotype, although not well known due to only a small number of reported cases worldwide, appears to be consistent with that seen in sporadic PD but with a slightly earlier age of onset.

Genes Associated with Autosomal Recessive Inheritance

Parkin (PARK2)

Parkin mutations are a major cause of early onset PD, possibly accounting for up to half of all cases presenting up to 45 years of age and a greater proportion (up to 77%) of those presenting before 30 years of age. *Parkin* has a role in maintenance of the intracellular ubiqutin/proteosome pathway involved in the degradation of proteins that otherwise accumulate to toxic levels. Unlike *LRRK2*- and *SNCA*-related PD, synuclein pathology is not seen at autopsy, although few brains have been systematically examined after death. Patients with *Parkin* mutations will often be well maintained on small doses of levodopa but experience prominent motor complications at an early stage. *Parkin* mutations should always be considered in patients presenting before the age of 45 years and in those presenting with lower limb dystonia, which may be present for years before emergence of classical parkinsonian symptoms.

PINK1 (PARK6)

Mutations in *PINK1* may account for up to 5% of cases of familial PD in Caucasian populations. *PINK1* and *Parkin* interact intracellularly to mediate the ubiquitination of mitochondrial substrates, required to facilitate the removal of damaged mitochondria. *PINK1* facilitates the movement of *Parkin* from the cell cytosol to damaged mitochondria. The clinical phenotype in *PINK1*-related PD is an early onset disease with a greater tendency to dystonia and neuropsychiatric complications than sporadic PD. A marked sleep benefit has also been reported in patients functioning with relative normality for hours in the morning before their first dose of levodopa.

DJ1 (PARK7)

DJ-1 may also play a role in mitochondrial function and may be linked in some way to the pathway involving *Parkin* and *PARK1*. Mutations in this gene account for approximately 1% of cases of familial PD. Ten mutations associated with PD have been described to date. The phenotype appears to be a slowly progressive one and shares features with *Parkin* and *PINK1* parkinsonism, with a good levodopa response and neuropsychiatric features.

APPROACH IN THIS CASE

The same important principles that apply to genetic testing for any condition apply in this case. Consideration must be given to (1) the likelihood of an underlying monogenic mechanism for the patient's presentation; (2) the potential for genetic testing to alter clinical management; (3) the value of a genetic diagnosis to the patient with respect to prognostication and family planning; and (4) the benefit to be derived, if any, from testing asymptomatic family members. In the case of this woman, with an onset in her late thirties and an affected father, there is a relatively high chance that a genetic cause for her presentation may be found. Her management will not be affected by a genetic diagnosis. Although one could say that caution with respect to levodopa-related motor fluctuations may be informed by a confirmed genetic diagnosis, one would always exhibit caution in prescribing levodopa in patients of this age group regardless, so management will not truly be affected.

Concerning the benefit to the patient, there is always value to be gained from having a genetic diagnosis in hand to explain to a patient why he or she developed a particular disease, and although potentially of no pragmatic benefit, most patients will place major emphasis on the importance of this information to them. This patient is unlikely to have children at age 42 years, so preconceptual counseling is not an issue. Her unaffected siblings should be formally counseled with respect to asymptomatic testing. I generally advise against such testing when there is a potential for nonpenetrance (as in *LRRK2*) and more important is the lack of useful disease-modifying intervention at this point in time should an asymptomatic carrier be identified. The societal and financial implications for mortgage applications and loan approval should also be taken into account, depending on the local legislation.

In this case, genetic testing in the patient after counseling is appropriate, and with a positive history of PD in her father, it is reasonable to start with *LRRK2* analysis. If a gene panel using next-generation sequencing is locally funded and available, this alternative simultaneously examines both dominant and recessive possibilities for a similar price to Sanger sequencing of individual genes. The clinical story is suggestive of a recessive PD, although the father's history points toward dominant inheritance. The father's diagnosis may be a red herring because the principle of the phenocopy is well described in studies of pedigrees with monogenic PD. Further complicating matters is the debated issue of *Parkin* mutations manifesting in heterozygous and compound heterozygous individuals.

KEY POINTS TO REMEMBER

- The identification of an underlying monogenic cause of PD in patients will have no impact on the management of their disease.
- The vast majority of patients who have a positive family history of PD will not have a pathological mutation in any of the known disease-causing genes discovered to date.
- Next-generation sequencing techniques offer a more cost-effective approach to pursuing genetic testing where indicated, screening a panel of genes associated with PD with a rapid turnaround time.

Further Reading

Kalinderi K, Bostantjopoulou S, Fidani L. The genetic background of Parkinson's disease: Current progress and future prospects. *Acta Neurol Scand* 2016 Feb 12. doi: 10.1111/ane.12563. [Epub ahead of print]

Kumar KR, Weissbach A, Heldmann M, et al. Frequency of the D620N mutation in VPS35 in Parkinson disease. *Arch Neurol* 2012;69(10):1360–1364.

Olgiati S, Quadri M, Bonifati V. Genetics of movement disorders in the next-generation sequencing era. *Mov Disord* 2016 Apr;31(4):458–470.

Polymeropoulos MH, Lavedan C, Leroy E, et al. Mutation in the alpha-synuclein gene identified in families with Parkinson's disease. *Science* 1997;276(5321):2045–2047.

Ross OA, Soto-Ortolaza AI, Heckman MG, et al. Association of LRRK2 exonic variants with susceptibility to Parkinson's disease: A case–control study. *Lancet Neurol* 2011;10(10):898–908.

8 "I Am Not Sure If I Should Do DaT"

Richard A. Walsh

You have been asked to see a patient who has been given a diagnosis of Parkinson's disease. The referring physician has performed some initial investigations that include magnetic resonance imaging (MRI) and an ioflupane (^{123}I) dopamine transporter scan (DaTscan). The reports confirm a structurally normal brain with evidence for "an asymmetrical reduction in radionucleotide uptake in the striatum on the left more than right, consistent with a diagnosis of early Parkinson's disease." While awaiting an appointment with you, a dopamine agonist was started, with no symptomatic benefit and prominent somnolence and postural dizziness as side effects. The patient had returned to his doctor, who had introduced levodopa, which had an immediate moderate effect on gait and general movement. However, by the time the appointment with you arrives, this benefit appears to have diminished. The patient and his wife are clearly concerned and want you to explain why the "best tablet" for Parkinson's disease is no longer effective.

What do you do now?

IMAGING THE NIGROSTRIATAL TRACT: CLINICAL UTILITY AND PITFALLS

The confirmation of Parkinson's disease (PD) remains a postmortem process, achievable only by the demonstration of the appropriate Lewy body pathology with a clinical story that is in keeping with it. In life, the absence of such a definitive diagnostic test is a well-worn lament, and efforts continue to identify a reliable and specific biomarker in PD, which includes an imaging biomarker of nigrostriatal denervation. For a diagnosis of PD to be made, the clinical examination remains the gold standard tool, which even in the hands of an experienced movement disorders neurologist can be wrong as often as 10% of the time. The absence of an objective test to make a diagnosis of PD is particularly felt in the research field, in which pathological heterogeneity has a potential to skew trial findings in the study of potentially useful neuroprotective agents that remain the holy grail of PD. On a practical level, an inability to give a definitive diagnosis to patients makes it difficult to accurately prognosticate or predict response to therapy.

Degeneration of nigrostriatal dopaminergic neurons can be linked to the evolution of the cardinal motor features of PD. Although invisible to conventional MRI and computed tomography (CT) imaging, this tract can be indirectly imaged using radiolabeled compounds, of which many are in use, that are taken up in the terminal junctions of these neurons in the dorsal (motor) striatum. The dopamine transporters (DaTs) are located presynaptically in this region and play a major role in the regulation of synaptic dopamine concentration within the striatum. Their location serves as a useful opportunity to assess the integrity of nigrostriatal neurons. Loss of DaT uptake can be interpreted as degeneration where there is no other confounding factor, such as drugs that may interfere with the interaction between radioligand and the DaT (Table 8.1). One of the most commonly employed presynaptic imaging techniques is single-photon emission computed tomography (SPECT) imaging using ^{123}I, such as the ^{123}I-fluoro-propyl-CIT scan, commercially available as a DaTscan (Fig. 8.1). Early changes in evolving PD include subtle asymmetry with loss of the putaminal "tail" signal on one side.

In general practice, dopamine transporter scans are not always available, and cost can be prohibitive where there is access. It is important to consider the urgency when ordering a dopamine transporter scan. Because PD is a slowly evolving disorder, there is almost always the luxury of time and a therapeutic trial to determine if the clinical course is in keeping with idiopathic PD. Importantly, DaT imaging will not indicate if a patient has typical or atypical parkinsonism. Nigrostriatal denervation is a feature of progressive supranuclear palsy and

TABLE 8.1 **Drugs That Can Interfere with Interpretation of a**
¹²³I-Fluoro-propyl-CIT Scan and Those That Need Not Be Stopped

Drug to Be Held (Timing of Cessation)	Drugs That Can Be Continued
Benztropine (3–5 days)	Levodopa
Buproprion (5–7 days)	Dopamine agonists
Hyoscine (5–7 days)	Trihexyphenidyl
Citalopram, escitalopram, and paroxetine (1 day)	Selegiline and rasagiline
Sertraline (3 days)	Propanolol and metoprolol
Modafinil (3 days)	Primidone
Cocaine (2 days)	Neuroleptics and other D2 antagonists
Fentanyl (1 day)	Amantadine

multiple systems atrophy, and DaT imaging will therefore be abnormal. One of the most common errors made is to send a patient to the nuclear medicine department for a scan with the question, "Typical or atypical parkinsonism?" However, there are four situations in which imaging of the nigrostriatal system is of value and can be justified.

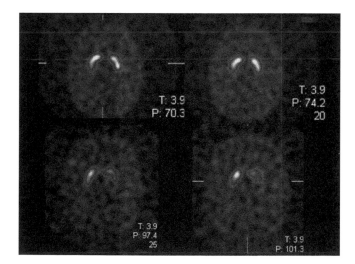

FIGURE 8.1 Dopamine transporter scans in a patient with essential tremor (top) and a patient with idiopathic Parkinson's disease (bottom) demonstrating the asymmetrical loss of the striatal "tail" on one side in keeping with early dorsal striatal degeneration.

In a Patient with Parkinsonism Who Is Being Treated with a D2 Receptor Antagonist

The most common situation in which this scenario occurs is when a patient with a primary psychiatric diagnosis, such as schizophrenia, is sent to the clinic by his or her psychiatrist with a unilateral tremor or a greater degree of brady-kinesia than would typically be anticipated in a drug-induced extrapyramidal syndrome. Most psychiatrists will be very familiar with the mild neuroleptic-related parkinsonian features that are common in patients taking these agents chronically at moderate or high doses. Referral for a movement disorders opinion is generally made when sensitivity to low neuroleptic doses is observed, when parkinsonian features have prominent asymmetry or tremor predominance, or when there is unexpected progression in the absence of a change in neuroleptic dose so that an opinion is sought. An added complexity that arises is the fact that these patients are often reliant on the neuroleptic in question for satisfactory management of their psychiatric condition, sometimes precluding cessation or reduction to determine to what degree the drug is the cause. The advice given is generally to switch to an alternative agent with less D2 antagonism, such as quatiapine or clozapine, but these agents have often been tried already, leaving no choice but to use an agent with greater risk of extrapyramidal side effects. On the rare occasion that a patient with parkinsonism is found to be on a drug that can be stopped completely, such as regular prochlorperazine or metoclopramide for nausea, it makes far more sense to stop the drug and determine if the parkinsonism gradually improves rather than perform an expensive scan. For patients for whom this is not possible, it is reasonable to perform a DaT scan, which should be normal in a drug-induced syndrome. A subset of these patients will have early unmasking of an evolving neurodegenerative syndrome by the D2 antagonist; parkinsonism that improves with cessation but does not resolve completely is not believed to be "tardive" parkinsonism as is seen with dystonia but more a reflection of this unmasking process.

Where Functional Parkinsonism Is Suspected

This clinical situation is truly quite rare but not unheard of. Patients presenting with functional parkinsonism will often have had exposure to the complex phenotype in another family member, providing some potential for modeling of symptoms. Some cases of functional unilateral resting tremor are not distractible or entrainable and therefore defeat the main clinical tools we rely on to determine if there is an organic component. Occasionally, other features, such as a reduced arm swing, stooped posture, and general bradykinesia, are not easily overcome using clinical maneuvers. The author has encountered a patient with a very accurate phenocopy of parkinsonism, including hypometric saccades, who was later found to have functional parkinsonism. In these occasional challenging cases, in which the clinical exam is not sufficient to make a positive diagnosis of a functional disorder, a DaT scan is a useful adjunct to reassure both the patient and the physician that the nigrostriatal dopaminergic system is intact.

In a Patient with Late-Onset Psychosis and Cognitive Impairment in Whom Dementia with Lewy Bodies Is Suspected

Colleagues in psychiatry will not infrequently ask for a neurology consultation on a patient with late-onset hallucinations or paranoia in the absence of any premorbid psychiatric diagnosis. This will often raise suspicion of an "organic" or secondary psychosis as opposed to a primary psychiatric diagnosis such as late-onset schizophrenia. It is now typical for immune-mediated neuropsychiatric conditions such as anti-voltage-gated potassium channel encephalitis and anti-NMDA receptor encephalitis to be considered. Given the rarity of these alternatives, it is more likely that a patient with these symptoms has an evolving dementia with Lewy bodies, particularly where sensitivity to neuroleptics has been demonstrated. In this situation, a DaT scan can a helpful way of identifying nigrostriatal denervation prior to the emergence of extrapyramidal signs.

The Monosymptomatic Tremor

Despite the very clear clinical difference between essential tremor and parkinsonian disorders, and most clinicians' confidence in their ability to identify PD over essential tremor clinically, there are always cases that defy easy classification. A typical situation is a patient who presents with an action tremor that has an additional rest component, in the absence of rigidity and where bradykinesia assessment is contaminated by tremor. Normal arm swing and good facial expression, which can be seen in tremor-predominant PD, can make the distinction between tremor-predominant PD and essential tremor challenging. In this situation, it is reasonable to institute a diagnostic trial of levodopa or other dopaminergic therapy to assess response. The introduction of levodopa without a firm diagnosis can be confusing for patients and can generate stress given its association with PD. In these cases, a DaT scan can be helpful in providing supportive data to allow patient reassurance or otherwise. Unfortunately, some patients will have a true "overlap" syndrome with both common diseases being present, making time and observation the best tools at the neurologist's disposal.

- Structural imaging of the brain in PD using conventional CT and MRI is typically normal and of little value when clinical features are otherwise typical.
- Radionucleotide imaging can be performed to assess the integrity of the nigrostriatal system. This is expensive and not routinely available, and it is incapable of reliably differentiating between typical and atypical forms of parkinsonism.
- An abnormal ^{123}I-fluoro-propyl-CIT scan (or DaTscan) is not pathognomonic for idiopathic PD; rather, it signifies loss of nigrostriatal neurons, which can be seen in a number of degenerative disorders with parkinsonism.
- The most common clinical situation in which dopamine transporter imaging is helpful is in the patient on neuroleptic therapy that cannot be stopped who has developed evolving parkinsonism. DaT imaging should be normal in drug-induced tremor.

Further Reading

Brigo F, Turri G, Tinazzi M. ^{123}I-FP-CIT SPECT in the differential diagnosis between dementia with Lewy bodies and other dementias. *J Neurol Sci* 2015;359(1–2):161–171.

Rodriguez-Porcel F, Jamali S, Duker AP, Espay AJ. Dopamine transporter scanning in the evaluation of patients with suspected parkinsonism: A case-based user's guide. *Expert Rev Neurother* 2016;16(1):23–29.

Scherfler C, Schwarz J, Antonini A, et al. Role of DAT-SPECT in the diagnostic workup of parkinsonism. *Mov Disord* 2007 Jul 15;22(9):1229–1238.

PART II

Atypical Parkinsonism

9 Parkinson's Disease with an Unusual Tremor

Richard A. Walsh

You are asked for a second opinion on a 62-year-old man with a 2-year history of Parkinson's disease diagnosed after he presented with imbalance causing falls, loss of facial expression, and difficulty with fine hand movements. He reports difficulty swallowing solids and complains of postural dizziness. He has prominent urinary urgency and frequency but no incontinence. He reports a complete absence of erections for 2 years. During the past 18 months, he has gone from independent ambulation to requiring a walking frame. His wife volunteers that he can strike out in his sleep. He has had no response to 900 mg levodopa daily and has not experienced dyskinesia. On examination, he has a high-pitched, breathy dysphonia. He has no rest tremor. With posture and action there are fine, irregular jerky movements of the digits on both sides. There is mild bilateral upper limb rigidity and bradykinesia. In the lower limbs there is a velocity-dependent catch at the knee in keeping with spasticity.

What do you do now?

MULTIPLE SYSTEM ATROPHY

When a patient presents with a prior diagnosis of Parkinson's disease (PD) but is not responding to treatment or is progressing rapidly, the first task is to look for the so-called "red flags" suggesting an alternative diagnosis. Because the diagnosis of PD is a clinical one, it is not uncommon for early uncertainty to exist before more discriminating clinical features appear. The most commonly encountered mimics of PD in this age group are multiple system atrophy (MSA), progressive supranuclear palsy (PSP), vascular parkinsonism, and dementia with Lewy bodies (DLB). Corticobasal syndrome, a clinical entity reflecting a disparate number of underlying pathologies, can also present with parkinsonism but is less common. All of these share a generally poor or short-lived response to levodopa, prominent gait disturbance with early falls, and a rate of deterioration that would be unusual in PD. Accuracy in the diagnosis of these atypical parkinsonian disorders is important to allow surveillance for complications specific to each disorder, to give patients and families a realistic impression of prognosis, and to allow appropriate enrollment to clinical trials.

The striking features of this patient's presentation are the rapidity of progression and the absence of a response to a relatively high dose of levodopa. Early falls can be seen in the first year in both PSP and MSA, but more commonly in PSP, where the falls are often backwards. Falls in the early years are not expected in treated PD. In this patient there is also a history of syncope, likely related to orthostatic hypotension. Early autonomic involvement is another important clue and should prompt consideration of MSA; although common also in PD and DLB, it is generally seen later in the disease course and to a milder degree in these disorders. Orthostatic hypotension can be a side effect of high-dose levodopa treatment, but when causing syncope there is generally additional dysautonomia. Symptomatic bladder disturbance is almost universal in MSA, and its absence should caution against the diagnosis. Similarly, the presence of normal erectile function in men in the first year of symptoms is unusual in MSA. The sleep disturbance reported here is suggestive of REM sleep behavior disorder and an underlying so-called "synucleinopathy" (i.e., parkinsonian disorders in which alpha-synuclein deposition is the pathological hallmark, such as PD, DLB, or MSA) rather than PSP (in which abnormal tau deposition is the underlying pathological change). Early cognitive impairment and hallucinations are not present here, making DLB unlikely. Therefore, on the basis of the history alone, the most likely clinical diagnosis in this case is atypical parkinsonism due to probable parkinsonian-predominant variant MSA (MSA-P) (Box 9.1).

BOX 9.1 **Gilman Consensus Criteria for a Clinical Diagnosis of MSA (1998)**

Definite MSA

Requires pathologic evidence of synuclein-positive glial cytoplasmic inclusions in the CNS with neurodegenerative changes in striatonigral or olivopontocerebellar structures.

Probable MSA

A sporadic, progressive, adult (>30 y)-onset disease characterized by:

- Autonomic failure involving urinary incontinence (inability to control the release of urine from the bladder, with erectile dysfunction in males) or an orthostatic decrease of blood pressure within 3 min of standing by at least 30 mmHg systolic or 15 mmHg diastolic *and*
- Poorly levodopa-responsive parkinsonism *or*
- A cerebellar syndrome

Possible MSA

A sporadic, progressive, adult (>30 y)-onset disease characterized by:

- Parkinsonism (bradykinesia with rigidity, tremor, or postural instability) *or*
- A cerebellar syndrome (gait ataxia with cerebellar dysarthria, limb ataxia, or cerebellar oculomotor dysfunction)
- At least one feature suggesting autonomic dysfunction (otherwise unexplained urinary urgency, frequency or incomplete bladder emptying, erectile dysfunction in males, or significant orthostatic blood pressure decline that does not meet the level required in probable MSA) *and*
- At least one of:

  - Babinski sign with hyperreflexia
  - Stridor
  - Possible MSA-P
  - Rapidly progressive parkinsonism
  - Poor response to levodopa
  - Postural instability within 3 y of motor onset
  - Gait ataxia, cerebellar dysarthria, limb ataxia, or cerebellar oculomotor dysfunction
  - Dysphagia within 5 y of motor onset
  - Atrophy on MRI of putamen, middle cerebellar peduncle, pons, or cerebellum
  - Hypometabolism on FDG-PET in putamen, brainstem, or cerebellum
  - Possible MSA-C
  - Parkinsonism (bradykinesia and rigidity)
  - Atrophy on MRI of putamen, middle cerebellar peduncle, or pons
  - Hypometabolism on FDG-PET in putamen
  - Presynaptic nigrostriatal dopaminergic denervation on SPECT or PET

The clinician should look for the following features of the history and exam specifically to help discriminate between the various forms of atypical parkinsonism.

Oculomotor Abnormalities

Hypometric saccades and a loss of smooth-pursuit eye movements are common to all forms of parkinsonism and are of no discriminating value. Square-wave jerks are seen more commonly in PSP than in MSA but can be seen in both disorders. Gaze-evoked nystagmus, as seen in this patient, and positioning downbeat nystagmus in particular (i.e., on performing the Hallpike–Dix maneuver), if present, are the more specific oculomotor features of MSA.

Atypical Tremor

Although a pill-rolling rest tremor typical of PD can be seen in MSA, most patients will present with an akinetic-rigid syndrome without tremor. There can be some diagnostic confusion where there is mini-polymyoclonus of the fingers that can mimic a tremor. The appearance is typically jerky and irregular, affecting individual fingers without any particular pattern. This can be stimulus sensitive and increases with action. Myoclonus with marked stimulus sensitivity can be seen in corticobasal syndrome.

Nocturnal Stridor

A history of nocturnal stridor should be sought if a bed partner is available because in the right clinical setting this is almost pathognomonic for MSA. Both vocal cord paralysis and adductor dystonia have been described. Some patients can have daytime stridor that can be particularly distressing and this is a poor prognostic indicator. Continuous positive airway pressure (CPAP) has been used with some success in small reported series, and in some cases a tracheostomy is undertaken for daytime stridor. Some bed partners also report an irregular pattern of breathing, including inspiratory sighs; these can also be present during waking hours and are an indication of central respiratory dysfunction, which can complicate the picture.

Orthostatic Hypotension

The absence of a history consistent with orthostatic hypotension should not be relied on. A proper assessment of lying and standing blood pressure for up to 3 minutes must be performed because asymptomatic changes are common. It is useful to look for an absence of a rise in pulse rate (in the range of 10–15 beats in normal individuals) as an additional sign of dysautonomia. Dysautonomia is common in DLB, but the extensive and sometimes profound involvement seen in MSA is quite specific.

Dystonia/Dyskinesia

Antecollis and levodopa-induced craniocervical dystonia are more commonly seen in MSA than in PD, affecting up to 50% of patients and often in the absence of any clinical benefit. Facial dyskinesia in the absence of dyskinesia elsewhere should also raise suspicion of MSA. The generalized choreiform levodopa-induced dyskinesias that are common with chronic treatment in PD are not typically seen in MSA. Dystonia affecting the upper or lower limbs can also be seen but is not useful as a specific diagnostic feature. Corticobasal syndrome is associated with asymmetrical upper limb rigidity and dystonia, with additional evidence of cortical sensory loss and dyspraxia helping to differentiate this syndrome from PD.

Pyramidal Signs

Brisk deep tendon reflexes and extensor plantar responses can be a feature of MSA. Lower limb spasticity should be differentiated from rigidity with its velocity dependence. It is always worth considering cervical pathology (e.g., from cervical spondylosis) in a patient with a gait disorder and pyramidal signs in the lower limbs.

Cognitive and Behavioral Changes

Although it was previously believed that cognitive impairment is uncommon in MSA, recent evidence suggests that frontal–subcortical cognitive dysfunction, similar to that seen in PSP, is not uncommon. Family members often identify behavioral changes. Emotional incontinence in particular can be a feature of MSA, with a greater tendency to become tearful. Pathological laughter can be seen in either MSA or PSP but is more common in the latter. It can be distressing to both patient and family. Early cognitive impairment is by definition a feature of DLB, although prominent hallucinations distinguish this from other forms of atypical parkinsonism with cognitive impairment.

Ataxia

MSA may present as an adult-onset sporadic gait ataxia (broad-based and unsteady), with cerebellar signs, milder parkinsonism, and autonomic dysfunction. This form of MSA is termed MSA-cerebellar (MSA-C).

INVESTIGATIONS

When available, patients with atypical parkinsonism should have magnetic resonance imaging (MRI) of the brain performed, which can be helpful in

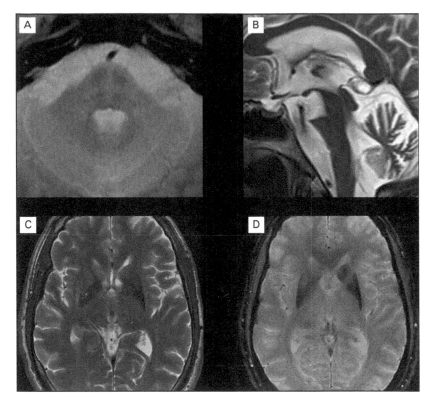

FIGURE 9.1 (A) Pontine atrophy and the "hot-cross bun" sign in MSA-C. (B) Sagittal T1 view of the brainstem in MSA demonstrating pontine atrophy. (C) Axial T2 view in MSA-P demonstrating left > right putaminal atrophy and a hyperintense putaminal rim. (D) Gradient echo sequence in MSA-P revealing hypointensity in the dorsolateral putamen.

demonstrating characteristic changes in MSA that are effectively diagnostic in the right clinical setting (Fig. 9.1). Gradient echo sequences can demonstrate hypodensity in the posterolateral aspect of the putamen, which can be supportive of a diagnosis of MSA and is usually seen with the parkinsonian-predominant variant (MSA-P). The specificity of this sign is greater when associated with putaminal atrophy. Axial T2-weighted sequences can demonstrate a corresponding hyperintense lateral putaminal margin. In MSA-C (cerebellar type), pontine and cerebellar atrophy is more prominent. Hyperintensity of the middle cerebellar peduncles (MCPs) and the "hot-cross bun" sign in the pons are not pathognomonic of MSA but support a clinical diagnosis. Hyperintensity of the MCPs can also be seen in the spinocerebellar ataxias and the fragile X tremor–ataxia syndrome.

Anal sphincter EMG has been used as a test to discriminate between MSA and PD but is not widely available. There appears to be a large range of normal physiological findings and considerable overlap between the PD and MSA populations studied. The test is probably most specific very early in the course of suspected MSA.

MANAGEMENT

Motor Features
Up to one-third of patients will have a response to levodopa lasting more than 2 years, but the gratifying response seen in PD is typically absent. It is worthwhile pushing the dose to at least 1200 mg/day (in three or four divided doses) before starting a downwards titration if there has been no discernable benefit. Notably, patients with MSA will often report feeling generally better on lower doses of levodopa, having experienced none of the motor benefit and all of the peripheral dopaminergic side effects (nausea and worsening postural hypotension) at higher doses. Amantadine is a reasonable second-line agent to which a minority of patients may respond to some degree. Side effects can be limiting, but the absence of any other viable symptomatic agent warrants a therapeutic trial of up to 300 mg/day.

In the absence of significant parkinsonism, as may be the case in MSA-C, there is no value in a trial of levodopa or amantadine. In the face of progressive disability due to ataxia or unresponsive parkinsonism, it is worthwhile to introduce the concept of using a wheelchair early. With a caregiver, this allows patients to maintain their mobility and ability to socialize. Walking frames can be impractical in these patients with significant upper limb disability.

Dystonia or facial dyskinesia can be treated with botulinum toxin injections.

Dysautonomia
Bladder dysfunction can sometimes be worsened by anticholinergics because patients with MSA will often have neurogenic outflow problems. Urodynamics and assessment by a urologist experienced in dealing with this disorder is valuable. Many patients with MSA undergo prostate surgery prior to diagnosis for seemingly obstructive symptoms. Some patients with adequate upper limb function perform self-intermittent catheterization; otherwise, a urethral or suprapubic catheter can be placed.

Orthostatic hypotension sometimes responds well to conservative measures such as raising the head of the bed to 30 degrees, increased fluid intake, and additional dietary salt. As mobility deteriorates, some patients will complain less of orthostatic symptoms as they spend more time in a sitting position due to increasing ataxia. Postural dizziness or even syncope can still be troublesome even when rising from a supine position in the morning. In these patients, treatment with fludrocortisone (0.1–0.3 mg/day; monitor electrolytes) can be effective. Midodrine is an alpha agonist that can also be helpful (2.5–10 mg TID). The use of these agents is complicated by supine hypertension, although in a disease with such a poor prognosis as MSA, this can sometimes be tolerated. Regular swallow assessment can minimize the risks of aspiration and pneumonia.

Other

When nocturnal stridor is present, CPAP is sometimes used to maintain airway patency. Daytime stridor is more concerning and is a poor prognostic indicator. Tracheostomy is sometimes considered. Importantly, these approaches do not reduce the risk of sudden death due to central ventilatory failure in these patients. The potential for respiratory arrest should be mentioned to allow discussion about invasive ventilation should this occur.

Patients with MSA and their families will require considerable assistance as the condition progresses. Involvement of the full multidisciplinary team is crucial, given the multiple issues and rapid progression. Social supports should be sought to reduce caregiver burden and maximize quality of life in the home for as long as practical.

KEY POINTS TO REMEMBER

- MSA is a cause of atypical parkinsonism that is characterized by early and prominent dysautonomia with a variable degree of cerebellar and extrapyramidal involvement.
- Progression, as a rule, is faster than seen in idiopathic PD, and response to levodopa is typically poor or short-lived. There is no role for a trial of levodopa where rigidity and bradykinesia are absent or contribute little to overall disability in MSA.
- MRI can be a useful tool in helping confirm a clinical suspicion of MSA. The typical changes described may not be apparent on an initial scan, so it is worth repeating imaging 1 or 2 years later if the clinical features and course are typical of MSA.
- MSA can present with asymmetrical parkinsonism with tremor and apparent levodopa responsiveness. The characteristic features sometimes may not be apparent until a number of years after initial symptom onset, explaining the often-delayed diagnosis of MSA.

Further Reading

Brown RG, Lacomblez L, Landwehrmeyer BG, et al. Cognitive impairment in patients with multiple system atrophy and progressive supranuclear palsy. *Brain* 2010;133(8):2382–2393.

European MSA Study Group. Presentation, diagnosis, and management of multiple system atrophy in Europe: Final analysis of the European multiple system atrophy registry. *Mov Disord* 2010;25(15):2604–2612.

Gilman S, Low P, Quinn N, et al. Consensus statement on the diagnosis of multiple system atrophy. *Clin Auton Res* 1998;8:359–362.

Lee JY, Yun JY, Shin CW, et al. Putaminal abnormality on 3-T magnetic resonance imaging in early parkinsonism-predominant multiple system atrophy. *J Neurol* 2010;257(12):2065–2070.

Quinn N. Multiple system atrophy—The nature of the beast. *J Neurol Neurosurg Psychiatry* 1989;52:78–89.

10 Falling All the Time

Richard A. Walsh

A 67-year-old retired teacher presents with a fall. His family recounts a recent history of recurrent backwards falls. Fifteen months after his first fall he was falling every week. His wife has noticed a change in his ability to perform manual tasks, writing in particular. He complains of difficulty reading and following the movement of the ball at football games. He has become more passive and withdrawn.

He enters your clinic room wearing sunglasses, in a wheelchair pushed by his wife. He has a prominent staring expression and square-wave jerks. Self-initiated vertical saccades are abnormal in range and velocity in both directions, improving with oculocephalic maneuvers. Horizontal saccades and pursuit eye movements are normal. Accommodation is poor. He has a gravelly dysphonia with features of a cerebellar dysarthria. Jaw-jerk is brisk. There is mild bilateral upper and lower limb bradykinesia and rigidity. Verbal fluency, abstraction, and Luria hand maneuvers are all impaired.

What do you do now?

PROGRESSIVE SUPRANUCLEAR PALSY

Although postural instability is one of the cardinal features of Parkinson's disease (PD), falls are uncommon in the first 5 years because much of the early gait impairment tends to be levodopa-responsive and the progression is slow. In advanced PD, non-levodopa-responsive gait abnormalities prevail and probably result from degeneration of nondopaminergic brainstem neurons with a specific role in locomotion and control of axial posture. A patient presenting with parkinsonism and early gait impairment with falls should raise the question of an atypical parkinsonism, in particular progressive supranuclear palsy (PSP). Vascular parkinsonism and multiple system atrophy (MSA) can also have a prominent gait component but not of the sort seen in PSP, in which axial rigidity, loss of safety awareness, and impulsivity combine with loss of postural reflexes to give rise to falls. The increasing availability of postmortem tissue in "brain banks" from patients with a clinical diagnosis of PSP is revealing that a number of different proteinopathies can give rise to a PSP-like syndrome, including corticobasal degeneration and Alzheimer's disease and even Creutzfeldt–Jakob disease. Even Whipple's disease can produce a syndrome mimicking PSP with a vertical gaze abnormality. Diagnostic criteria for PSP are given in Box 10.1. The National Institute of Neurological Disorders and Stroke (NINDS) criteria are stringent and like most criteria are aimed at specificity rather than sensitivity. It is now recognized that there is huge variability in the clinical presentation of PSP and many, and perhaps a majority, of pathologically confirmed cases would not meet formal criteria early on in the disease, thus highlighting the diagnostic challenge.

CLINICAL PHENOTYPES IN PROGRESSIVE SUPRANUCLEAR PALSY

A number of phenotypic variants associated with PSP pathology have been described.

Richardson's Syndrome

This is the classical syndrome described in eight patients by Steele, Richardson, and Olszewski in 1963. The clinical picture is of an akinetic rigid syndrome with prominent postural instability, axial rigidity, and a vertical gaze palsy, much like that described in this case. Retrospective clinicopathological correlations now question the primacy of this phenotype among the others described next, at least in the first 2 to 3 years of symptoms.

National Institute of Neurological Disorders and Stroke Diagnostic Criteria for PSP

Definite Progressive Supranuclear Palsy

Clinically probable or possible PSP and histopathologic evidence of typical PSP

Probable Progressive Supranuclear Palsy

- Gradually progressive disorder
- Onset at age 40 or later
- Vertical supranuclear palsy and prominent postural instability with falls in the first year of disease onset
- No evidence of other diseases that could explain the foregoing features, as indicated by mandatory exclusion criteria

Possible Progressive Supranuclear Palsy

- Gradually progressive disorder
- Onset at age 40 or later
- Either vertical supranuclear palsy or both slowing of vertical saccades and prominent postural instability with falls in the first year of disease onset
- No evidence of other diseases that could explain the foregoing features, as indicated by mandatory exclusion criteria

Supportive Features

- Symmetric akinesia or rigidity, proximal more than distal
- Abnormal neck posture, especially retrocollis
- Poor or absence of response of parkinsonism to levodopa therapy
- Early dysphagia and dysarthria
- Early onset of cognitive impairment including at least two of the following: apathy, impairment in abstract thought, decreased verbal fluency, use of imitation behavior, or frontal release signs

Exclusion Criteria

- Recent history of encephalitis
- Alien limb syndrome, cortical sensory deficits, focal frontal or temporoparietal atrophy
- Hallucinations or delusions unrelated to dopaminergic therapy
- Cortical dementia of Alzheimer type
- Prominent early cerebellar symptoms or prominent early unexplained dysautonomia
- Severe, asymmetric parkinsonian signs
- Neuroradiologic evidence of relevant structural abnormalities
- Whipple's disease, confirmed by polymerase chain reaction

Progressive Supranuclear Palsy with Parkinsonism

Presentation with a parkinsonian syndrome of asymmetrical bradykinesia and rigidity and tremor, with or without oculomotor abnormalities, is common. Lack of levodopa responsiveness and rate of change over time with a slow drift toward a syndrome more similar to the more classical Richardson's syndrome may ensue.

Pure Akinesia with Gait Freezing

This is a distinct phenotype that is more closely linked to true PSP pathology than some of the other phenotypes discussed here, which are more often mimicked by other non-PSP pathologies. Early and prominent postural instability and freezing of gait can be present for more than 5 years before the more typical cognitive, parkinsonian and eye movement features emerge. Disease duration is also different, with it being common for patients to survive beyond 10 years from the initial diagnosis.

Progressive Supranuclear Palsy–Corticobasal Syndrome

The distribution of tau pathology in some patients favors a frontoparietal cortical syndrome in keeping with a corticobasal syndrome with an asymmetrical parkinsonism with dystonia and cortical sensory loss. This can be indistinguishable from the other 4R tauopathy corticobasal degeneration, which accounts for approximately 50% of patients with corticobasal syndrome. Further demonstrating the complexity of clinicopathological correlation in neurodegenerative disease, corticobasal degeneration pathology can also give rise to a PSP-like syndrome.

Progressive Supranuclear Palsy–Progressive Nonfluent Aphasia

Presentations within the spectrum of frontotemporal dementia are also seen with PSP pathology confirmed postmortem. A speech disorder characterized by early and prominent apraxia of speech with hesitancy, agrammatism, and phonemic errors has been proposed as a subtype of PSP.

EYE MOVEMENTS IN PROGRESSIVE SUPRANUCLEAR PALSY

The clinical feature best recognized in PSP is the vertical supranuclear gaze palsy described by Steele, Richardson, and Olszewski, who provided the first clinicopathological description of this syndrome in 1964. It is important to pay close attention to oculomotor function when confronted with any patient with parkinsonism. Eye movements should be reassessed over time because not all patients will have clinically evident abnormalities at presentation. A supranuclear gaze palsy manifests as a reduction in the velocity and range of voluntarily initiated vertical saccades with normal oculocephalic reflexes. Abnormalities of downward saccades are more specific for PSP because limitation in the upward direction develops normally with age. A mistake made by less experienced examiners is to assess vertical pursuit eye movement only. Early in the course of the disease, the range of movement on pursuit can be normal, with vertical slowing evident only with saccadic testing that assesses the fastest form of eye movement, thus exposing subtle abnormalities. Horizontal eye movements are also affected in PSP, but later and less severely than those in the vertical plane.

Another mistake that can be made when testing vertical saccades is to ignore the potential for involuntary persistence of ocular fixation that gives the impression of impaired vertical gaze. This type of fixation is seen in disorders involving the frontal lobes and can therefore be seen in PSP, but it can also be seen in any other basal ganglia disease with frontal lobe involvement. For this reason, avoid sitting directly in the line of sight of the patient when testing eye movements. Where more subtle clinical changes are present, testing optokinetic nystagmus (OKN) with an OKN tape or drum can be a useful additional examination. Saccadic abnormalities can have important functional significance, as in this patient's case, for example when moving from one line of text to the next. Other ocular features in PSP are given in Box 10.2.

OTHER MOTOR FEATURES IN PROGRESSIVE SUPRANUCLEAR PALSY

Careful examination of the head and neck is important in patients with suspected PSP. Frontalis or procerus muscle overactivity (possibly dystonic) can lead to a startled or frowning appearance. Prominent nuchal rigidity is common but not specific for PSP. This nuchal rigidity can make it difficult to test oculocephalic reflexes in practice. Some patients will have dystonic hyperextension

---

BOX 10.2   **Ocular Symptoms and Signs Seen in PSP Patients**

Vertical supranuclear gaze palsy
Blepharospasm or "apraxia" of eyelid opening
Square-wave jerks
Nystagmus
Limitation of ocular convergence
Eyelid retraction producing the characteristic expression
Photophobia

of the neck, which can sometimes cause significant pain. Botulinum toxin can sometimes be useful in this situation. Pyramidal tract signs are seen in approximately one-third of patients. The pseudobulbar speech disturbance in PSP is characterized in classical cases by a low-pitched, growling, spastic dysarthria with monotonous, ataxic features. A pseudobulbar dysarthria is also common, and most patients will require dietary modification at some stage of the disease because of dysphagia. Micrographia can be striking in PSP, and this can sometimes be a useful, albeit nonspecific, differentiating feature from PD, particularly if severe early in the course of symptoms. Freezing of gait is common in PSP as part of the prominent gait disorder.

COGNITION IN PROGRESSIVE SUPRANUCLEAR PALSY

The pseudobulbar affect in PSP is characterized by emotional incontinence and pathological laughter without mirth that can be distressing to both caregivers and patients. Some patients will have moaning or groaning episodes. The pattern of cognitive impairment in PSP is a frontal–subcortical dementia with variable involvement of linguistic, attentional, and memory functions. Perseveration, apathy, and disinhibition can also be observed. The "applause" sign has been described in PSP as a manifestation of frontal–subcortical dysfunction, but again it is a nonspecific feature. The patient is asked to clap three times as quickly as possible after demonstration by the examiner. A response with more than three claps is considered abnormal. Although previously thought to be a useful discriminating test, relatively recent reports suggest that it can be seen in other neurodegenerative diseases with prominent basal ganglia involvement as well as in Alzheimer's disease. Dyspraxia can be a feature of PSP and depends on the extent and distribution of cortical pathology. It is typically mild and bilateral but can be unilateral and more severe in keeping with a clinical diagnosis of a corticobasal syndrome.

INVESTIGATIONS

Magnetic resonance imaging (MRI) of the brain can be supportive where a clinical diagnosis of PSP is being considered. The typical appearance of tegmental midbrain atrophy seen on sagittal MRI sequences with relative preservation of pontine volume has been described as the "hummingbird" or "emperor penguin" sign (Fig. 10.1A). On the same sequences, the superior surface of the midbrain can have a concave appearance due to atrophy. On axial cuts, this midbrain atrophy has been likened to the bloom of a morning

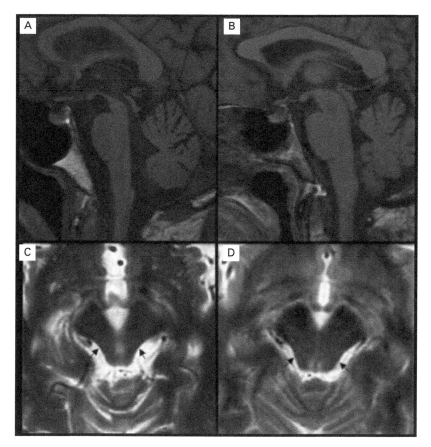

FIGURE 10.1 Sagittal T1-weighted MRI sequence demonstrating the hummingbird sign in progressive supranuclear palsy (A) compared to a healthy patient (B) and axial T2 image of the brainstem in PSP (C) demonstrating the "morning glory" sign produced by dorsolateral midbrain atrophy (black arrows) compared to a normal midbrain (D).

glory flower (Fig. 10.1B). The third ventricle is typically enlarged with concave walls. In some cases, atrophy of the superior cerebellar peduncles can be appreciated, although in practice this is difficult to appreciate. Gradient echo sequences are typically normal. Variable degrees of frontal cortical atrophy can be seen.

MANAGEMENT

In general, levodopa is unhelpful in PSP. A trial of levodopa may be warranted where the parkinsonism is causing significant disability and, as seen in multiple system atrophy, a minority of patients may experience a transient benefit. As with MSA, if no benefit is obtained after escalation to doses of 200 mg three times daily, it is reasonable to reduce to zero or to a level below which there is a clear deterioration. Amantadine can be tried for freezing and gait, with close attention paid to the possibility of cognitive deterioration to which these patients are particularly vulnerable. There has been interest in deep-brain stimulation of the pedunculopontine nucleus for postural impairment in PD, but this remains an unproven approach. Blepharospasm and "apraxia" of eyelid opening respond to botulinum toxin, with the more gratifying response being seen in blepharospasm. Artificial tears may help to avoid exposure keratitis and ease the discomfort associated with reduced blink frequency. Blue-tinted lenses are anecdotally of particular benefit for the photophobia in PSP, although in practice most patients will report benefit from standard sunglasses.

Selective serotonin reuptake inhibitors can be used for emotional apathy, depression, and pseudobulbar crying. The high risk of falling in addition to the poor judgment and disinhibition that can be a feature of the frontal-predominant dementia in these patients make safety an important consideration. Close supervision of patients at home is required. The manner in which some patients with PSP launch themselves out of a chair has been described as the "rocket" sign and is often accompanied by a tendency to fall backwards into a chair en bloc, with the risk of missing the target or banging their heads off the wall if not knocking the chair over completely.

Involvement of a multidisciplinary team is important. It should include a speech and language therapist, occupational therapist, and physiotherapist. Palliative neurology is a growing subspecialty and serves these patients well by addressing those issues for which there is no useful disease-modifying therapy. Information on local support groups should be provided to the patient and family to help them manage what is a rapidly progressive and very challenging disease for which there are currently no useful interventions.

KEY POINTS TO REMEMBER

· Progressive supranuclear palsy is best considered a syndrome that has been linked with heterogeneous pathological substrates, including the classical 4R tauopathy of PSP. This same PSP pathology has a diverse clinical spectrum, which continues to expand as our knowledge of the disease expands.
· Spend time on examining ocular signs, which can be of a very high yield when considering atypical parkinsonian syndromes.

- Midbrain atrophy on MRI can be a helpful but nonspecific imaging feature when considering PSP in a patient with parkinsonism, with midbrain tegmental atrophy giving rise to the "hummingbird" or "Emperor penguin" sign on sagittal midbrain views.
- A trial of levodopa and amantadine is still warranted in patients in whom PSP is suspected, although the response is generally poor or short-lived and early discontinuation where benefit is lacking is advised.
- Patients should be encouraged to use a wheelchair early when falls become frequent. Although many patients will be reluctant to "give in" to this, it can be rewarding in allowing greater freedom of movement outside the home and easing the burden on carers.

Further Reading

Goetz CG, Leurgans S, Lang AE, Litvan I. Progression of gait, speech and swallowing deficits in progressive supranuclear palsy. *Neurology* 2003;60(6):917–922.

Lang AE. Clinical heterogeneity in progressive supranuclear palsy: Challenges to diagnosis, pathogenesis and future therapies. *Mov Disord* 2014 Dec;29(14):1707–1709.

Litvan I, Campbell G, Mangone CA, et al. Which clinical features differentiate progressive supranuclear palsy (Steele–Richardson–Olszewski syndrome) from related disorders? A clinicopathological study. *Brain* 1997;120:65–74.

Respondek G, Stamelou M, Kurz C, et al. The phenotypic spectrum of progressive supranuclear palsy: A retrospective multicenter study of 100 definite cases. *Mov Disord* 2014 Dec;29(14):1758–1766.

Steele JC, Richardson JC, Olszewski J. Progressive supranuclear palsy. *Arch Neurol* 1964;10:333–359.

Williams DR, de Silva R, Paviour DC, et al. Characteristics of two distinct clinical phenotypes in pathologically proven progressive supranuclear palsy: Richardson's syndrome and PSP–parkinsonism. *Brain* 2005:128(6):1247–1258.

11 "My Arm Is Not Working"

Robertus M. A. de Bie and
Susanne E. M. Ten Holter

You see a 63-year-old man with a 3-year history of difficulty with his left arm. It began with a sensation of pins and needles and lack of coordination. His handwriting became unreadable, and over time he was unable to use his arm at all. In the last few months there have also been involuntary movements over which he has no control. He tells you that "it is like the arm has a will of his own." Clinical findings are posturing of the left hand with flexion of the wrist in rest, rigidity of the left arm, and weakness of the left hand. There are rapid jerky movements of the left arm when making a movement and upon tactile stimulation. When asked to demonstrate a task with his left hand, such as brushing his teeth, he keeps staring at his hand without it making a proper movement. The patient has no problems performing tasks with his right hand. Cranial nerves, deep tendon reflexes, and plantar responses are normal. There is tactile extinction and dysgraphesthesia in the left hand.

What do you do now?

CORTICOBASAL SYNDROME

The lack of control over his left arm and the spontaneous movements are compatible with an alien limb phenomenon. There is also dystonia, stimulus-sensitive myoclonus, cortical sensory loss, and ideomotor dyspraxia. This combination of a progressive asymmetrical movement disorder and higher cortical dysfunctions is suggestive of a corticobasal syndrome (CBS).

CBS is an atypical parkinsonian syndrome, characterized by a slowly progressive marked asymmetrical movement disorder presenting in one limb (mostly an arm) with a variety of potential associated clinical motor and cognitive features. The symptoms eventually spread to the contralateral arm or the ipsilateral leg.

Motor Features

The most common motor features are asymmetric bradykinesia, rigidity, postural instability, dystonia, tremor, and myoclonus. The tremor is often a "jerky" postural and action tremor. A tremor at rest is rare. Myoclonus is stimulus sensitive and elicited by voluntary actions, which are characteristics compatible with a cortical origin.

Sensory Features

If there is sensory impairment, it predominantly concerns cortical sensory loss. Examples are tactile extinction, astereognosis, and dysgraphesthesia. Cortical sensation can only be tested if primary sensation (e.g., touch, vibration, and pain) is intact. Testing tactile extinction should be done by administering simultaneous stimuli on both the left and the right side. Stereognosis can be tested by placing an object, such as a key or coin, in the patient's hand and asking the patient to name the object without actually seeing it. Graphesthesia can be tested by "writing" a number or letter on the palm and asking the patient to identify it.

Higher Cortical Features

Because the examination of higher cortical deficits can be challenging, this is addressed in more detail. One of the higher cortical features typical for CBS is dyspraxia. Dyspraxia is an impairment to carry out a skilled movement although the patient appears to understand the assignment. The inability may not be due to weakness, ataxia, or a sensory deficit. There are different types of dyspraxia. In ideomotor dyspraxia, the patient is unable to imitate a task upon instruction even though he or she understands the request. Ideomotor dyspraxia of the limb is a typical finding, but orofacial or truncal ideomotor dyspraxia can also occur. In ideational dyspraxia, the patient is not able to formulate and execute a task due to impaired conceptional knowledge. This type of dyspraxia is not typical for CBS and is more often seen in Alzheimer's disease, although it has been described in late-stage CBS as well. The dyspraxia can be apparent in daily activities or only upon testing. Evaluating dyspraxia requires a specific approach when examining a patient and should include the following:

- Imitation of a movement performed by the examiner
- Portraying a verbal demand using both a simple task (wave goodbye) and a sequence of movements (lighting a candle with a match)
- Matching tools and objects (nail and hammer) and using a tool correctly (telephone)

Although frequently associated with CBS, the alien limb phenomenon is not a pathognomonic sign. An alien limb phenomenon can also occur following a focal lesion (e.g., stroke or tumor) or after a corpus callostomy. In the literature, the alien limb phenomenon is sometimes classified into two variants: the anterior variant, with callossal and frontal (supplementary motor area, cingulate cortex, and medial prefrontal cortex) involvement, and the posterior variant (posterolateral parietal cortex, occipital cortex, and thalamus). Pathological and functional magnetic resonance imaging (MRI) studies suggest a bihemispherical or interhemispherical network disconnection. The alien limb phenomenon most often presents as an alien hand and predominantly on the nondominant side, but features can also appear in a leg. There is no clear-cut definition of the phenomenon, and the clinical presentation can vary. The patient should be aware of the movement without being able to control it. It can appear to the patient as if someone else controls the body part. The movement should also be directed to a specific task or goal, excluding nonspecific movements such as tremor, myoclonus, or dystonia. A manifestation can be grasping upon visual or tactile stimuli. Self-directed grasping can also occur. Often it is difficult to release the object, and the patient may need to use the other hand to do so. Another manifestation is intermanual conflict, in which purposeful movements of the "healthy limb" are counteracted by the alien limb. An example is taking off a sock that has just been put on, but very often these movements are not very specific. At the same time, the patient has difficulty initiating an intentional movement with the hand. Unintentional withdrawal can also occur. Groping is thought to be a frontal sign, intermanual conflict a callosal sign, and withdrawal a parietal sign, but often there is a mixture of features and a correct localization is difficult. The alien limb phenomenon can present with bizarre behavior, and it is important to recognize it is a symptom of cerebral pathology rather than to misinterpret it as a functional neurological disorder. As in this case, patients with CBS can also complain of a "useless limb" without it being an alien limb phenomenon, for example, due to dyspraxia.

Another higher cortical feature is dysphasia. This can be present in a broad spectrum from mild impairment to progressive nonfluent aphasia or mutism. Recently, it has become clear that CBS is also accompanied by early cognitive and neuropsychiatric deficits, such as general cognitive impairment, behavioral changes, and depression.

Etiology

The cortical basal syndrome can have different etiologies. Corticobasal degeneration (CBD) is well known. Other possible underlying pathologies are Alzheimer dementia (AD), frontotemporal lobe degeneration (FTLD), progressive supranuclear palsy (PSP), and Creutzfeld–Jacob disease. There are no specific clinical symptoms to determine the underlying pathology of CBS; therefore, the term CBD should be used only for the postmortem pathology diagnosis and the term CBS for the clinical diagnosis.

CORTICOBASAL DEGENERATION

Specific pathologic features of CBD include asymmetrical cortical atrophy (frontoparietal and frontotemporal) and degeneration of basal ganglia. Microscopically, ballooned achromatic cells are seen with an abnormal accumulation of tau protein in neurons and glial cells and astrocytic plaques. CBD is a sporadic neurodegenerative disease in the tauopathy family, which also includes AD, FTLD, and PSP. The onset of symptoms is in late adulthood, and a positive family history is rare. The mean age of survival is 7–9 years.

The corticobasal syndrome is the most common phenotypic presentation of CBD. Recently, three other clinical phenotypes of CBD have been described: the frontal behavioral–spatial syndrome, the nonfluent/agrammatic variant of primary progressive aphasia, and the progressive supranuclear palsy syndrome (PSPS). A summary of the features of these different phenotypes, as proposed by Armstrong and colleagues, is shown in Box 11.1.

DIAGNOSTICS

As noted previously, CBD is a pathological diagnosis. There are no diagnostic options to distinguish CBD from other etiologies of CBS. A treatable cause should be excluded. Routine blood, urine, and cerebrospinal fluid (CSF) tests are normal. There is currently no biomarker in CSF or blood available for CBD.

Features of the Different Phenotypes of Corticobasal Degeneration

Probable corticobasal syndrome including two of the following:

- Limb rigidity or akinesia
- Limb dystonia
- Limb myoclonus

And two of the following:

- Orobuccal or limb dyspraxia
- Cortical sensory deficit
- Alien limb phenomena (more than simple levitation)

Possible corticobasal syndrome including one of the following:

- Limb rigidity or akinesia
- Limb dystonia
- Limb myoclonus

And one of the following:

- Orobuccal or limb dyspraxia
- Cortical sensory deficit
- Alien limb phenomena (more than simple levitation)

The frontal behavioral–spatial syndrome including two of the following symptoms:

- Executive dysfunction
- Behavioral or personality changes
- Visuospatial deficits

The nonfluent/agrammatic variant of primary progressive aphasia with effortful agrammatic speech and at least one of the following:

- Impaired grammar/sentence comprehension with relatively preserved single-word comprehension
- Groping
- Distorted speech production (apraxia of speech)

PSPS including three of the following:

- Axial or symmetric limb rigidity or akinesia
- Postural instability or falls
- Urinary incontinence
- Behavioral changes
- Supranuclear vertical gaze palsy or decreased velocity of vertical saccades

Regarding the recent discoveries of paraneoplastic and autoimmune syndromes due to anti-neuronal antibodies, paraneoplastic screening should be considered in specific cases—for example, if there is a short history with rapidly progressive disease. Computed tomography or MRI should be performed to rule out a structural lesion. Findings of asymmetrical prominent atrophy of the corpus callosum, cerebral peduncles, or basal ganglia are reported and could be suggestive of CBD; however, their presence or absence has no influence on the clinical diagnosis of CBS. Ligand-based nuclear imaging is a subject of research that may present as a promising diagnostic tool for CBD in the future. Evoked potentials can vary from a normal signal to an abnormal asymmetrical response. Similar responses, however, have been described in other atypical parkinsonian disorders. Electroencephalogram (EEG) can also show a variety of findings from a normal EEG to nonspecific delta slowing or dysrhythmic signals. Electrophysiological diagnostics therefore have no role in the differentiation of CBD from other differential options. Because CBD is often accompanied with cognitive and neuropsychiatric disturbances a neuropsychological examination could be considered.

THERAPY

There are no therapeutic options to reverse or slow the neurodegenerative process. Symptomatic therapy to treat the symptoms should be attempted but tends to be disappointing. A levodopa trial is often tried, titrated up to 900–1200 mg a day for at least 1 month. There is often a limited response, and if a significant improvement is seen for a longer period of time, the diagnosis of CBD must be reconsidered. Treatment of myoclonus and dystonia could be more successful. Improvement of myoclonus has been reported with valproic acid, clonazepam, and levetiracetam. Dystonia can be treated with botulinum toxin injections. The most beneficial treatment is supportive therapy including physical therapy, speech therapy, and occupational therapy, preferably in a multidisciplinary setting in which experience of atypical parkinsonian disease is available.

KEY POINTS TO REMEMBER

- In the case of a progressive asymmetrical movement disorder with higher cortical dysfunction, always consider the possibility of CBS.
- When confronted with a patient with higher cortical dysfunction, specific assessment for dyspraxia, sensibility, and cognition is indicated.

- Corticobasal syndrome can have a variety of underlying pathologies.
- Corticobasal degeneration can have a number of different phenotypes.

Further Reading

Armstrong MJ, Litvan I, Lang AE, et al. Criteria for the diagnosis of corticobasal degeneration. *Neurology* 2013;80:496–503.

Chahine LM, Rebeiz T, Rebeiz JJ, Grossman M, Gross RG. Corticobasal syndrome: Five new things. *Neurol Clin Pract* 2014;4:304–312.

Grijalvo-Perez AM, Litvan I. Corticobasal degeneration. *Semin Neurol* 2014;34:160–173.

Sarva H, Deik A, William, Severt WL. Pathophysiology and treatment of alien hand syndrome. *Tremor Other Hyperkinet Mov (NY)* 2014;4:241.

12 "I See Them Sitting on My Bed, Doctor"

Susan H. Fox and Marina Picillo

A 75-year-old man with a 2-year history of cognitive decline is referred to your clinic by his family physician. The family's main concern relates to behavioral disturbances that started approximately 1 year ago. He has been experiencing well-formed visual hallucinations of people in his house, often at night when in low-level lighting in his bedroom. His wife reports that he has limited insight, with fear that thieves may be entering the house to steal their possessions. He also accuses her of infidelity. According to the man's wife, his cognitive state fluctuates significantly during the day, sometimes appearing very lucid. During the past few months he has also had slowness of general movement (e.g., walking and dressing). On examination he is hypomimic, bradyphrenic, and presents with symmetrical rigidity and slowness of movement. His past medical history is unremarkable apart from a diagnosis of REM sleep behavior disorder 6 years ago.

What do you do now?

DEMENTIA WITH LEWY BODIES

The clinical syndrome of a progressive cognitive decline giving rise to new functional dependence for activities of daily living is in keeping with a diagnosis of dementia clinically. Dementia can be due to a variety of underlying pathophysiological causes (Box 12.1). The presence of severe behavioral disturbance (e.g., delusions), hallucinations, and spontaneous parkinsonism in a patient with a prior history of REM sleep behavior disorder (RBD) should prompt the clinician to suspect a diagnosis of dementia with Lewy bodies (DLB), which represents the third most common cause of dementia (5%). However, other causes should be taken into account in the differential diagnosis. Alzheimer's disease (AD) is the most common form of dementia (50–75%) and typically presents with short-term memory problems, difficulty in recognizing familiar faces (prosopagnosia), and spatial disorientation. Parkinsonism and hallucinations may be present in the late stage of the disease. Vascular dementia is the second most frequent cause (20%) and is strongly suggested when there is either a temporal association of cognitive deficits with stroke or evidence of cerebrovascular disease on examination and imaging. Early language or behavioral symptoms should raise the question of frontotemporal lobar degeneration (<5%), which is characterized by younger age at onset and often associated with parkinsonism and positive family history. When assessing a patient with dementia and parkinsonism for the first time, a clinician should also consider the diagnosis of Parkinson's disease with dementia (PDD). As a rule of thumb, if dementia occurs more than 1 year after a clinical diagnosis of PD, the patient is considered affected by PDD. Where dementia occurs before or during the first year of a parkinsonian syndrome, the diagnosis is considered to be DLB. Despite this somewhat arbitrary distinction, the clinical manifestations of DLB and PDD reflect a common pathobiology (i.e., cortical Lewy bodies), thus the term Lewy body disease has been proposed as an umbrella term encompassing PD, PDD, and DLB.

BOX 12.1 **Most Common Diseases to Be Considered in the Differential Diagnosis of Dementia Syndrome**

1. Alzheimer's disease
2. Vascular dementia
3. Dementia with Lewy bodies
4. Frontotemporal lobar dementia
5. Parkinson's disease with dementia

Investigations

When evaluating a patient with progressive cognitive decline the first step is to rule out the presence of systemic processes, such as metabolic disturbances (e.g., hypothyroidism) and vitamin deficiency (e.g., vitamins B_6 and B_{12}). Assessing the patient's cognitive status is the next step. The Montreal Cognitive Assessment Scale can be used for screening (a score <26 is considered abnormal) and should be followed by a formal cognitive testing where available. Brain computed tomography/magnetic resonance imaging scan is helpful because certain imaging features may suggest a specific diagnosis (e.g., vascular lesions support a vascular dementia, and medial temporal lobar atrophy is suggestive of AD).

Cognitive Profile

The cognitive profile of DLB comprises both cortical and subcortical impairments with substantial attentional deficits and prominent executive and visuospatial dysfunction. As opposed to AD, memory impairment is not prominent in the early stages and may appear later as the disease progresses. Pronounced day-to-day and hour-to-hour fluctuations of cognition from clear thinking to drowsiness and lethargy are considered a core feature of DLB. Diagnostic criteria for DLB are given in Box 12.2.

Hallucinations and Delusions

Visual hallucinations are recurrent and complex, tend to be formed, and are detailed involving anonymous or familial people and animals, usually insects; they are one of the most useful signposts to a clinical diagnosis of DLB. Some patients may also experience other sensory modalities hallucinations (i.e., tactile and auditory). Delusions (i.e., false beliefs) are usually paranoid and may include fear of intruders and spousal infidelity. Frightening hallucinations with severe paranoid delusions and agitation may lead to psychotic episodes that represent a common movement disorders emergency. In such cases, psychosis may be paradoxically exacerbated by neuroleptics. Thus, a positive history of severe neuroleptic sensitivity is strongly suggestive of DLB.

Parkinsonism

Spontaneous parkinsonism is one of the core features of DLB. Bilateral rigidity, slowness of movements, and postural instability are typical, and tremor is less common. Levodopa responsiveness is variable but is certainly less than in PD. Take care when a patient is on treatment with typical neuroleptics as parkinsonism may be drug-induced.

BOX 12.2 **Criteria for the Clinical Diagnosis of Dementia with Lewy Bodies**

1. *Central feature* (essential for a diagnosis of possible or probable DLB)

   Dementia defined as progressive cognitive decline of sufficient magnitude to interfere with normal social or occupational function.

   Prominent or persistent memory impairment may not necessarily occur in the early stages but is usually evident with progression.

   Deficits on tests of attention, executive function, and visuospatial ability may be especially prominent.

2. *Core features* (two core features are sufficient for a diagnosis of probable DLB, one for possible DLB)

   Fluctuating cognition with pronounced variations in attention and alertness

   Recurrent visual hallucinations that are typically well formed and detailed

   Spontaneous features of parkinsonism

3. *Suggestive features* (if one or more of these is present in the presence of one or more core features, a diagnosis of probable DLB can be made. In the absence of any core features, one or more suggestive features is sufficient for possible DLB. Probable DLB should not be diagnosed on the basis of suggestive features alone.)

   REM sleep behavior disorder

   Severe neuroleptic sensitivity

   Low dopamine transporter uptake in basal ganglia demonstrated by SPECT or PET imaging

4. *Supportive features* (commonly present but not proven to have diagnostic specificity)

   Repeated falls and syncope

   Transient, unexplained loss of consciousness

   Severe autonomic dysfunction (e.g., orthostatic hypotension, urinary incontinence)

   Hallucinations in other modalities

   Systematized delusions

   Depression

   Relative preservation of medial temporal lobe structures on CT/MRI scan

   Generalized low uptake on SPECT/PET perfusion scan with reduced occipital activity

   Abnormal (low uptake) MIBG myocardial scintigraphy

   Prominent slow wave activity on EEG with temporal lobe transient sharp waves

5. A diagnosis of DLB is *less likely*

   In the presence of cerebrovascular disease evident as focal neurologic signs or on brain imaging

   In the presence of any other physical illness or brain disorder sufficient to account in part or in total for the clinical picture

   If parkinsonism only appears for the first time at a stage of severe dementia

Other Clinical Features Common in Patients with Lewy Body Dementia

RBD manifests with vivid dreams during REM sleep, without the physiological muscle atonia. Patients therefore act out their dreams, moving around the bed, vocalizing and shouting during the night, falling out of bed, or injuring themselves or their bed partner. The history is often obtained from the bed partner, who may report a long-standing history of sleep disorders prior the onset of dementia. RBD is frequently associated with all the Lewy body disorders (idiopathic PD and multiple system atrophy).

Severe autonomic dysfunction may occur early in the disease, producing orthostatic hypotension, cardiovascular instability, urinary incontinence, as well as constipation and impotence. Autonomic dysfunction may also contribute to repeated falls and syncope and the transient losses of consciousness that are seen in some patients with DLB. Depression as well as apathy and other behavioral issues are common complaints of the carers of these patients.

MANAGEMENT AND PRACTICAL ISSUES

In a patient presenting a sudden worsening of cognition, the first step is to rule out systemic processes (i.e., infections, metabolic issues, and vitamin deficiency). Furthermore, clinicians should always check the medication lists of such patients in order to limit non-essential drugs and avoid compounds potentially worsening cognitive functions (i.e., anticholinergics, benzodiazepines, tricyclic antidepressants).

Evidence indicates improvements with donepezil and rivastigmine for cognition, hallucinations, delusions, and activities of daily living without worsening of parkinsonism. Memantine appears to be well tolerated but provides modest benefits to patients. Hallucinations and delusions require treatment with atypical neuroleptics, with quetiapine being the first-line treatment. Clozapine may be even more effective but is considered second-line treatment due to the risk of idiosyncratic reactions (i.e., agranulocytosis) requiring weekly blood monitoring for the first 3 months and monthly thereafter. Atypical neuroleptics must be avoided due to the neuroleptic sensitivity reactions, which are characterized by the acute onset or exacerbation of parkinsonism and impaired consciousness. ECG is suggested prior to commencing these medications because DLB patients are at higher risk of developing autonomic and cardiac side effects.

Parkinsonism may benefit from levodopa, which should be administered with low doses and a slow titration because it can worsen hallucinations as well as cognitive and behavioral disturbances. For such a reason, dopamine agonists should be avoided.

Caregivers have to cope with the hallucinations and behavioral symptoms as well as with motor impairment that accompany LBD and are indeed more pronounced than in AD. From a practical standpoint, clinicians can advise to ensure enough lighting at night to reduce visual hallucinations. Furthermore, poor community awareness and the lower incidence of DLB compared to AD often mean that caregivers experience social isolation. Accessible, high-quality information and both instrumental and emotional social support should be offered to people with DLB and their families beginning in the diagnostic period. Families can contact AD associations for caregiver support and information about local instrumental support (e.g., daytime care services or any aid provided by the local health system).

KEY POINTS TO REMEMBER

- DLB is characterized by cognitive decline, hallucinations, behavioral disturbances (delusions), and parkinsonism.
- DLB has to be considered in the differential diagnosis of dementia syndromes as well as parkinsonian syndromes.
- Hallucinations and behavioral disturbances represent a major burden for caregivers and need to be managed.

Further Reading

McKeith IG, Dickson DW, Lowe J, et al. Diagnosis and management of dementia with Lewy bodies: Third report of the DLB Consortium. *Neurology* 2005;65(12):1863–1872.

Stinton C, McKeith I, Taylor JP, et al. Pharmacological management of Lewy body dementia: A systematic review and meta-analysis. *Am J Psychiatry* 2015;172(8):731–742.

PART III

Other Gait Disorders

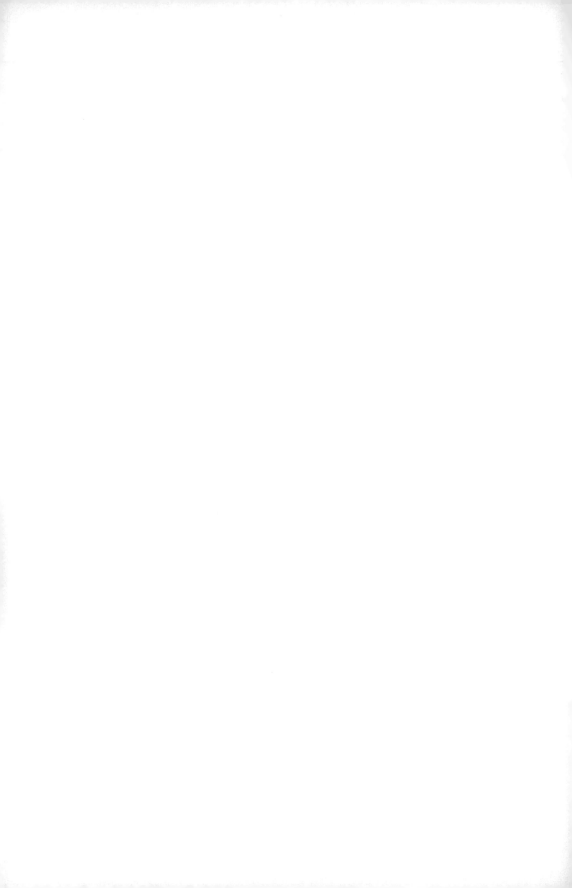

13 A New Loss of Order

Richard A. Walsh

You assess a 53-year-old man with a 2-year history of a slowly progressive gait disorder. He is a nonsmoker and rarely drinks alcohol. He has no known family history of note. He gradually became aware of the need to walk along walls for fear of falling. He did not fall spontaneously until 6 months after onset, but for the past 6 months he has had increasing falls. He is aware of a change in his speech and is concerned that people think he is drunk. He has mild dysphagia. Manual dexterity has deteriorated, but he remains independent.

On examination he has a scanning dysarthria. There is a tongue tremor on protrusion. He has a symmetrical intention tremor with dysmetria in the upper limbs. Dysdiadochokinesis is more prominent on the left side. Mild rigidity is present with coactivation in the upper limbs. Finger movements are slow without decrement. He has moderate heel–shin ataxia. Deep tendon reflexes are brisk, and sensory testing is normal. His gait is broad-based with a cane.

What do you do now?

ACQUIRED CEREBELLAR ATAXIA

The ataxias are a heterogeneous group of often uncommon diseases characterized by a predominance of cerebellar features. This is a vast and sometimes intimidating group for the general neurologist having insufficient experience to recognize some of the rarer syndromes, in particular the ever-expanding list of hereditary ataxias. A commonsense approach, however, should allow diagnosis of the most common and potentially treatable forms of acquired ataxia and will channel resources toward the more "high-yield" investigations including genetic testing where appropriate.

The ataxias can be broadly divided into three categories: (1) acquired ataxias due to nongenetic causes, (2) hereditary ataxias, and (3) neurodegenerative ataxias without evidence of heritability. Information gained from the family history, age of onset, rate of progression, and associated clinical features make it possible to devise a list of the most likely causes, although more than one-third of patients will have no diagnosis after investigation or an adult-onset sporadic ataxia of unknown etiology. As always, consideration of potentially treatable disorders should be at the forefront of the diagnostic process (Table 13.1). Some of the key discriminating clinical features are discussed next.

Age of Onset

Early onset ataxias develop before the age of 25 years and are most often due to metabolic or genetic disorders. Where genetic, early onset ataxias are typically recessively inherited and progress faster and are more disabling than late-onset forms. Late- or adult-onset ataxia is more likely to be acquired or degenerative, although with greater availability of genetic testing late-onset variants of hereditary ataxia are increasingly recognized. It is therefore important, however, to be aware of the evolving phenotypic picture of late-onset variants of the recessive ataxias seen in childhood.

Rate of Progression

Acute presentations should be worked up for a possible vascular, inflammatory (e.g., demyelination), or infectious (e.g., Epstein–Barr virus-associated cerebellitis) etiology (Fig. 13.1). Subacute onset of ataxia can be seen in toxic or nutritional disorders. Alcohol is a still a commonly encountered cerebellar toxin, and chronic alcoholic cerebellar degeneration can present rapidly in the event of a metabolic decompensation, particularly when there is a coexistent thiamine deficiency. This is sometimes seen in patients who have a background of alcohol dependence syndrome who are fasting or unable to eat due to surgery,

TABLE 13.1 **Forms of Potentially Treatable Adult-Onset Ataxia**

Cause	Treatment
Multiple sclerosis	Intravenous steroid if acute cerebellar lesion, although most commonly seen as a complication of progressive disease for which there is no useful intervention at this time
Steroid-responsive encephalopathy associated with autoimmune thyroiditis	Intravenous methylprednisolone
Cerebrotendinous xanthomatosis	Bile salts
Wernicke's encephalopathy	High-dose intravenous thiamine
Drug toxicity (e.g., lithium, phenytoin, metronidazole)	Cessation of the offending drug
Sensory ataxia secondary to B_{12} deficiency mimicking a cerebellar ataxia	Intramuscular vitamin B_{12} loading followed by 1000 µg oral B_{12} daily or intramuscular monthly
"Gluten ataxia"	Trial of coeliac diet for 6 months
Vitamin E deficiency	Vitamin E replacement
Ataxia secondary to anti-GAD antibodies	Trial of steroids, immunoglobulin, or plasma exchange
Paraneoplastic ataxia	Treatment of underlying malignancy; success more likely where antibodies are to cell-surface antigens

abdominal pathology, or other illness. The opportunity to treat thiamine deficiency presenting with ataxia as part of a Wernicke's encephalopathy must never be missed, although reversal of the chronic cerebellar changes is not to be expected. Acquired immune-mediated ataxic disorders or Creutzfeldt–Jakob disease (CJD) can also progress rapidly. Immune-mediated disorders include steroid-responsive encephalopathy associated with autoimmune thyroiditis (SREAT) and anti-GAD antibody-associated ataxia, both of which can respond to high-dose intravenous steroids. Anti-thyroid autoantibodies are not uncommon, and the patient who is being treated for presumed SREAT but failing to respond should be re-evaluated for an alternative diagnosis. CJD can mimic SREAT with prominent myoclonus, hallucinations, and rapidly developing cognitive impairment. Paraneoplastic cerebellar degeneration is rapidly

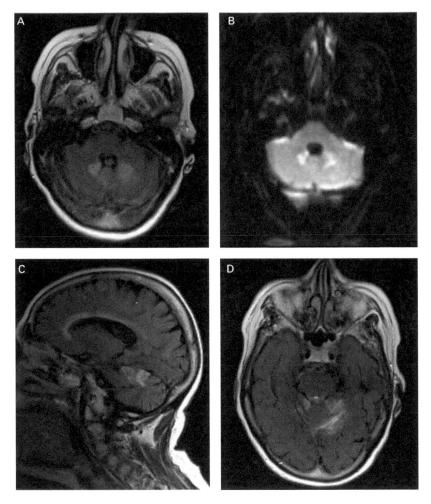

FIGURE 13.1 MRI images from a patient presenting with acute-onset ataxia including axial T2 (A and D), diffusion-weighted (B), and sagittal T1 (C) sequences, demonstrating acute cerebellar infarction in the territory of the superior cerebellar artery bilaterally.

progressive, can predate a diagnosis of cancer, and is associated with thymoma lung, breast, and ovarian malignancies.

Family History

Although at first an individual with ataxia may appear to have a sporadic or acquired disorder, it is not uncommon for other affected family members to have gait difficulties, dismissed as being alcohol-related or due to "rheumatism." As always, great care should be taken when obtaining the family history. Furthermore, the absence of a positive family history does not preclude a diagnosis of an autosomal dominant ataxia, but testing would typically be directed at acquired or degenerative disorders first, as well as consideration of the recessive ataxias, which are a less common cause of late-onset ataxia.

MRI Findings

Magnetic resonance imaging (MRI) is mandatory where available, given its ability to narrow the diagnostic possibilities. It can reveal immediately if there is an acquired structural cause for ataxia such as a posterior fossa tumor, cerebellar stroke, or Arnold–Chiari malformation. Cerebellar atrophy is the most common finding in general, and this can be isolated or associated with other imaging clues. Conversely, in the early stages of Friedreich's ataxia, a normal-appearing cerebellum is expected, so a normal scan does not preclude a genetic form of ataxia. Bilateral T2 hyperintensities involving the middle cerebellar peduncles (MCPs) are seen in fragile X tremor ataxia syndrome (FXTAS) but also in multiple system atrophy (MSA) and often unilaterally and more discrete in multiple sclerosis. In MSA with predominant parkinsonian features (MSA-P), the addition of gradient echo sequences is invaluable to identify hypointensity in the lateral putamen caused by iron deposition. MSA or the cerebellar subtype (MSA-C) is associated with the "hot-cross bun" appearance on MRI as well as bilateral hyperintensities of the MCPs, indistinguishable from FXTAS. The latter, however, is typically associated with subcortical white matter changes that are not expected in MSA. Gradient echo MRI sequences also reveal the linear hypointensity around the brainstem structures seen in superficial siderosis (Fig. 13.2) and the basal ganglia iron deposition in the neurodegenerative diseases associated with brain iron accumulation (NBIA). In rapidly progressive ataxias it is important to include diffusion-weighted MRI sequences because it is on these sequences that the basal ganglia hyperintensities seen in CJD are most prominent.

Associated Clinical Features

Sometimes the cerebellar features are so prominent that more subtle additional signs can be overlooked. Fundoscopy and examination of the palate are often the first casualties. Although it is rare to find any significant abnormality, the presence of retinal pigmentation (mitochondrial cytopathy, SCA-7) or a palatal tremor (adult-onset Alexander disease) can be helpful. Check the Achilles tendon for a tendon xanthoma for the same reason. Look for pyramidal signs that might raise suspicion of multiple sclerosis. Orthostatic hypotension may be the only clinical feature revealing a diagnosis of MSA and can frequently be asymptomatic. The stigmata of excessive alcohol consumption should also be

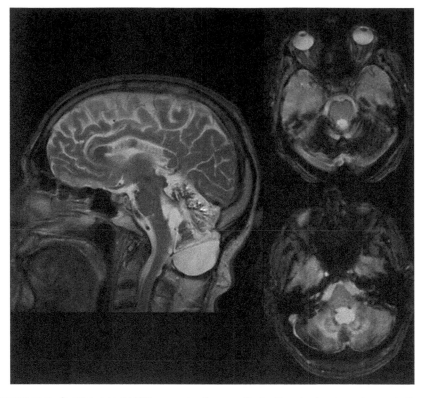

FIGURE 13.2 Sagittal and axial MRI sequences from a patient with a slowly progressive cerebellar syndrome and hearing loss following posterior fossa surgery, demonstrating sagittal T2 and gradient echo hypointensity surrounding the midbrain in keeping with superficial siderosis.

sought routinely because stated intake is often far from the truth. Peripheral neuropathy is more common in the recessive ataxias. If there is marked impairment of dorsal column function, vitamin B_{12} levels should be checked. Spasticity in the lower limbs can be seen in MSA.

DIAGNOSIS

The adult-onset sporadic ataxic syndrome described in this patient is a predominantly cerebellar one with additional parkinsonism. Brisk lower limb reflexes suggest pyramidal involvement. Parkinsonism and ataxia can be seen in FXTAS and the spinocerebellar ataxias (SCAs; SCA-2 and SCA-3), where it can be levodopa-responsive, although the absence of a family history is against these (although not to the point of exclusion). The normal sensory examination makes a sensory ataxia unlikely. It is likely that we are dealing with a "central"

TABLE 13.2 **Acquired Adult-Onset Cerebellar Syndromes**

Etiology	Diagnostic Test
Toxic/metabolic	
Alcoholic cerebellar degeneration	Anterior–superior vermial atrophy on MRI
Drugs (phenytoin, valproate, lithium)	Drug history
Neuroferritinopathy	MRI brain (with gradient echo sequences)
Nutritional/endocrine	
Thiamine deficiency	Thalamic and mammillary hyperintensity on MRI
Vitamin E deficiency	Vitamin E levels
Hypothyroidism	TSH and T4
Hypo/hyperparathyroidism	Cerebellar and cerebral calcification on computed tomography
Vascular	
Cerebellar stroke	MRI of brain
CNS vasculitis	MRI of brain, angiography, CSF analysis
Autoimmune/inflammatory	
"Gluten ataxia"	Anti-celiac antibodies
Autoimmune cerebellar ataxia	Anti-GAD antibodies
Steroid Responsive Encephalopathy Associated with Autoimmune Thyroiditis (SREAT)	Anti-thyroperoxidase antibodies, CSF analysis
Demyelinating/multiple sclerosis	MRI of brain, CSF oligoclonal bands
Sarcoidosis	Chest x-ray, CSF analysis, serum calcium and ACE
Related to underlying malignancy	
Primary cerebellar malignancy	MRI brain
Metastatic malignancy	MRI brain
Paraneoplastic or autoimmune syndrome	Anti-Hu, -Yo, -Ri, -Tr, -mGluR1, and anti-VGKC antibodies

(*continued*)

TABLE 13.2 **Continued**

Etiology	Diagnostic Test
Degenerative	
Multiple system atrophy	MRI brain ("hot-cross bun" sign in cerebellar variant)
Infective or transmissible	
CJD	MRI brain, CSF 14-3-3 protein, EEG
Viral cerebellitis	CSF viral PCR and serum IgM/IgG titers
Structural	
Arnold–Chiari malformation	MRI brain

ACE, angiotensin-converting enzyme; CJD, Creutzfeldt–Jakob disease; CNS, central nervous system; CSF, cerebrospinal fluid; EEG, electroencephalogram; MRI, magnetic resonance imaging; PCR, polymerase chain reaction; TSH, thyroid-stimulating hormone.

cerebellar ataxia, either a primary cerebellar disease or cerebellar dysfunction as part of a more widespread neurological disorder. Tongue tremor is generally uncommon in hereditary ataxic syndromes but can be a useful feature to note in possible MSA, although this is not a specific sign. With the additional suggestion of dysautonomia, given the bladder dysfunction and the mild symmetrical rigidity, MSA-C is near the top of our differential diagnostic list and an MRI with gradient echo sequences is most helpful in this setting. Some neurologists will use anal sphincter electromyography as a diagnostic test in MSA to demonstrate the autonomic involvement with denervation of Onuf's nucleus. However, the specificity of this test, which is unpleasant for patients, is questionable.

A balance must be reached between avoiding an excessive amount of tests at the first visit and bringing patients back every 6 months for investigations in a piecemeal fashion. Where imaging is not diagnostic, a positive family history suggesting either dominant or recessive inheritance should trigger a preliminary search for genetic forms of ataxias based on the most common forms or specific clinical features. If the clinical suspicion for a genetic form of ataxia remains high, testing should be performed even with a negative family history.

Many neurologists will start with more basic biochemical and imaging testing while other investigations are awaited. Routine testing of thyroid function, B_{12}, immunoglobulins, low-density lipoprotein, alpha-fetoprotein, albumin, and vitamin E is not unreasonable given the relatively minor cost of these tests. A second tier can include autoantibodies (anti-GAD antibodies, anti-tissue transglutaminase antibodies, and anti-thyroperoxidase antibodies) and a "paraneoplastic panel" searching for the less common acquired ataxias, although these will be checked first if clinical suspicion exists (Table 13.2). Cerebrospinal fluid (CSF) examination should also be performed where there is a possibility of an autoimmune etiology (cells and oligoclonal bands), prion disease (14-3-3 protein), or superficial siderosis (xanthochromia).

KEY POINTS TO REMEMBER

- All patients presenting for the first time with a cerebellar syndrome should have an MRI performed.
- Place a priority on excluding the treatable causes of ataxia, however uncommon.
- Avoid mistaking cerebellar slowing with true parkinsonian bradykinesia, which is marked by decrement and fatigability on finger-tapping.
- The absence of a family history does not exclude a genetic form of ataxia.
- Search closely for associated clinical clues other than ataxia that might improve the diagnostic yield, which can be frustratingly low in these disorders.

Further Reading

Galvin R, Bråthen G, Ivashynka A, et al. EFNS guidelines for diagnosis, therapy and prevention of Wernicke encephalopathy. *Eur J Neurol* 2010;17:1408–1418.

Gilman S, Wenning GK, Low PA, et al. Second consensus statement on the diagnosis of multiple system atrophy. *Neurology* 2008;71:670–676.

Klockgether T. Sporadic ataxia with adult onset; Classification and diagnostic criteria. *Lancet Neurol* 2010;9:94–104.

Van Gaalan J, van de Warrenburg B. A practical approach to late-onset cerebellar ataxia: Putting the disorder with lack of order into order. *Pract Neurol* 2012;12:14–24.

14 Falls

Susan H. Fox

A 79-year-old man is referred with progressive slowness over a few years, and he was noted to take longer walking on the golf course. During the past few months, he had fallen many times trying to turn round in his bathroom and kitchen. His daughter was very concerned because he was also more forgetful. She thought he may have hit his head during one of the falls. He is on medications for high blood pressure, and he is an ex-smoker. On examination, he has bruising on his forehead and face; he has some difficulty with recent memory. He has a positive glabellar reflex; cranial nerve examination is normal. He has some mild rigidity in both legs with generally slower movements of foot tapping. Cerebellar testing and also power and sensory testing are normal. He is able to stand unaided but with a wide base. He has hesitation on starting to walk and then, once walking, his stride is short steps and a wide base; he has normal arm swing. He is unable to turn without freezing and overbalancing, and he has to be helped back to the room.

What do you do now?

CAUSES OF FALLS IN THE ELDERLY

Falls in the elderly are multifactorial and may not always be due to neurological problems. Further details on the history and examination need to be determined to exclude any of these causes. Thus, the following should be determined: significant postural changes in blood pressure (BP) measurements (including lying BP, standing BP, BP after 5–10 minutes, and BP after walking), visual acuity and the presence of cataracts, joint pain and deformity, and a clear history that falls were not triggered by obstacles and mechanical falls.

Non–neurological Reasons for Elderly People Falling

- Medications—many drugs cause nonspecific dizziness, sedation, etc.
- Syncope—or presyncope due to cardiac disease, medication, dehydration, etc.
- Visual—many reasons for reduced ability to see (e.g., cataracts and macular degeneration)
- Musculoskeletal—joint disease affecting hips and knees with pain and stiffness and "mechanical falls"
- Fatigue

All such causes were effectively ruled out in this patient. The additional clinical findings also suggest a more specific possible neurological cause.

SPECIFIC NATURE OF THE GAIT DISORDER THAT IS CAUSING FALLS

Determination of the neurological cause of falls is aided by watching the person walk. If the person cannot walk unaided, then note the level of assistance required to support the person (e.g., ranging from non-weight-bearing to the use of walls and the amount of cane use). If possible, try to assess the patient walking without a cane or walker and have someone walk with him or her for support—to enable arm movements to be seen. There are several phases to the gait assessment; all parts can help in determining the cause. Observe the patient getting up from the sitting position, stand, walk approximately 10 m down an unobstructed corridor, turn, and come back (if possible):

- Getting up from the chair—needs to use arms to get up or able to get up without help; impulsively jumps up
- Posture when standing—look from side and back
- Starting off/gait initiation—freezing/start-hesitation

- Stride—length of steps, pace/speed; width of base; arm swing present and symmetrical and in keeping with stride length length
- Posture when walking—does it change?
- Abnormal movement in limbs or legs when walking
- Turning in a semicircle; number of steps should be less than two or three
- Postural reflexes with the "pull" test (quick tug standing behind subject, allow one or two steps of retropulsion, and be prepared to catch the person)
- Tandem gait (walk heel–toe) for ataxia; with wall to aid if required
- Rhomberg's—distinguishes cerebellar from sensory ataxia (patient stands with feet together and closes eyes—positive test in sensory ataxia is increased sway with eyes closed compared to open and indicates sensory loss via dorsal columns; in cerebellar ataxia, closure of eyes makes no difference to degree of sway)

In this patient, the important clinical features include some freezing when starting to walk (start hesitation) and short steps with relatively normal arm swing and some associated rigidity and slowness in the legs, suggesting "lower body" parkinsonism. Normally, the arm swing is in keeping with stride length (e.g., small steps are usually accompanied by an absent or reduce arm swing and are suggestive of parkinsonism). In this case, a "normal" arm swing may actually be "abnormal" and suggests a frontal lobe gait disorder; sometimes such conditions are associated with an exaggerated arm swing. The wide-based gait is not due to cerebellar ataxia because there is no evidence of cerebellar disease on testing, and sensory testing is also normal. The other reason for a wide-based gait is so-called gait apraxia. This is a term used to describe difficulty walking, despite normal motor and sensory function, and it generally implies higher cortical dysfunction (e.g., frontal/parietal lobe). The patient also has a positive glabellar tap (repetitive tapping of the nose and asking the patient not to blink but blinking occurs), which is a nonspecific signs for frontal–striatal/basal ganglia pathology. Thus, a positive glabellar tap is not specific for Parkinson's disease (although classically described in this condition); rather, it can be present in conditions associated with frontal lobe disease. Other so-called frontal-release signs may be useful to elicit, including testing for paratonia (moving the limb and feeling for resistance associated with the patient "helping you"); positive jaw jerk; and primitive reflexes such as grasp reflex, pout, snout, and palmomental reflexes. In this patient, brisk reflexes are also significant and indicate likely frontal motor cortex involvement. Overall the findings point to diffuse pathology (i.e., symmetrical signs) within frontal/prefrontal cortex and/or subcortical basal ganglia circuits.

WHAT IS THE MOST LIKELY PATHOLOGY CAUSING THIS TYPE OF GAIT DISORDER?

The first test is a brain MRI. If this does not show any abnormality, order a CT brain scan because rarely brain calcification can cause a similar clinical picture—so-called Fahr's disease. Full cognitive testing is also useful to assist in localizing the lesion as well as defining the degree of cognitive impairment, which is likely in these disorders. Cognitive issues—especially impulsivity and lack of judgment and awareness of risks—contribute to increased risks of falls.

Pathological Causes of Gait Apraxia

- Diffuse cerebrovascular disease—most common cause; diffuse small vessel disease and lacunar infarcts affecting centrum semiovale and periventricular frontal lobe and interconnecting corpus callosum. Commonly the degree of vascular changes seen on brain imaging may not correlate with clinical disability.
- Normal pressure hydrocephalus—should always be considered as a diagnosis because it may be amenable to surgery with ventriculoperitoneal shunting and improved gait if treated early enough. The gait apraxia is due to secondary compression of frontal cortex from the expanding of ventricles, and the syndrome of normal pressure hydrocephalus classically presents with the triad of gait apraxia, urinary symptoms, and cognitive impairment. The diagnosis, however, is notoriously difficult, and there are no clinically available standards tests that are specific (e.g., testing cerebrospinal fluid removal to determine a benefit of shunting is unreliable). In the elderly, this is often overdiagnosed due to the common feature of enlarged ventricles but often with concomitant brain atrophy. If surgery is contemplated, risks of the procedure need to be carefully evaluated.
- Progressive supranuclear palsy (PSP)—pure akinesia type; rare presentation of PSP with gait apraxia and early falls, before classical eye and bulbar signs appear.
- Corticobasal syndrome—rarely causes gait apraxia; more commonly asymmetrical arm apraxia.

- Bilateral striopallidodentate calcinosis (Fahr's disease)—rare cause of gait apraxia; can be familial or sporadic presentation and usually presents earlier in life than in this patient (i.e., in the 40s and 50s). Brain CT shows extensive bilateral calcifications in the dentate nuclei of the cerebellum and basal ganglia. In general, there is progressive neurologic dysfunction with cognitive and basal ganglia symptoms (parkinsonism and gait disorder but also hyperkinetic movements). Other causes of calcification have to be excluded, such as biochemical abnormalities and the absence of an infectious, traumatic, or toxic cause.

In this patient, extensive periventricular and frontal white matter disease was reported on the brain MRI due to vascular disease. There was dilatation of the ventricles, but this was in keeping with the degree of atrophy. He had no intracranial issues due to the falls; always check for coexistent subdural hematomas in elderly with repeated falls. The final diagnosis of gait apraxia due to chronic vascular disease was made. This was likely due to chronic hypertension. Cognitive testing reported cognitive impairment and frontal and parietal dysfunction, and a diagnosis of vascular dementia was also made.

MANAGEMENT OF PATIENT

The main aim is education to prevent falls and reduce ongoing pathology. Managing vascular risk factors is important, including BP control. It is not clear if aspirin and lowering cholesterol have an impact on preventing gait worsening in these patients. However, referral to stroke prevention clinics is useful for expert guidance. No pharmacological treatments have a major impact on this type of gait disorder. Management remains supportive, and fall prevention is the prime focus of care. The patient and family should be counseled that the risk of falling is very high. Early preventative use of a wheelchair is advised. Exercising within safety limits is important.

KEY POINTS TO REMEMBER

- There are many causes of falls in the elderly. Simple at-home occupational therapy assessments are useful for reducing the risk of mechanical falls.
- To date, no pharmacological therapies prevent falls, and in general, drugs will cause more side effects than benefit.
- Falls prevention clinics and other physiotherapy-led groups are useful as an educational setting for patients and families.

Further Reading

Callisaya ML, Srikanth VK, Lord SR, et al. Sub-cortical infarcts and the risk of falls in older people: Combined results of TASCOG and Sydney MAS studies. *Int J Stroke* 2014 Oct;9(Suppl A100):55–60.

Fleischman DA, Yang J, Arfanakis K, et al. Physical activity, motor function, and white matter hyperintensity burden in healthy older adults. *Neurology* 2015 Mar 31;84(13):1294–1300.

Gillespie LD, Robertson MC, Gillespie WJ, et al. Interventions for preventing falls in older people living in the community. *Cochrane Database Syst Rev* 2012 Sep 12;9:CD007146.

Snijders AH, van de Warrenburg BP, Giladi N, et al. Neurological gait disorder in elderly people; Clinical approach and classification. *Lancet Neurol* 2007;6:63–74.

15 Siblings with Instability

Richard A. Walsh

A 57-year-old man meets you for the first time. He has
a late-onset cerebellar ataxia with a similarly affected
sister and unaffected parents when they died at 72 and
61 years of age. He had been attending a colleague
for many years until their retirement, and despite
numerous investigations he remains undiagnosed. On
a review of his records you find that a comprehensive
metabolic screen was performed that was unrevealing.
Cerebrospinal fluid analysis was unremarkable. Magnetic
resonance imaging of brain in this man and his sister
revealed marked cerebellar atrophy. Structural imaging
was otherwise normal apart from mild frontal atrophy.

On examination he has a mild cerebellar dysarthria.
There is downbeat nystagmus in the primary position and
on horizontal gaze. He has moderate dysdiadochokinesia
with intention tremor in the upper limbs bilaterally. Lower
limb reflexes are brisk and there is a mild catch bilaterally.
Plantar responses are extensor. He has a spastic ataxia,
walking with a frame.

What do you do now?

GENETIC TESTING IN HEREDITARY CEREBELLAR ATAXIA

Any patient presenting with a cerebellar syndrome should have the benefit of a thorough search for acquired and reversible forms of ataxia, which although admittedly rare, take precedence over genetic testing. Once a broad biochemical screen has been sent, and has returned normal or negative, the question of a degenerative or heredodegenerative ataxia is often next to be considered. Slowly evolving syndromes, like that of the patient depicted here, and particularly those with a suggestion of a family history, are more likely to fit into the heredodegenerative category. Genetic testing typically follows where available, although not all clinicians will have access to this. For those who do have access, the process of selecting individual genes to sequence has not always been a straightforward one, particularly with respect to rare syndromes with unfamiliar phenotypes. Furthermore, the cost-effectiveness of some tests selected without a huge degree of supportive clinical data or familiarity is questionable. With the advent of next-generation sequencing, however, there has been an explosion of diagnostic potential and an opportunity to provide patients with a diagnosis where in the past they relied on a generic diagnostic label of "ataxia."

WHERE DO I START?

A sensible starting point when considering any potentially genetic syndrome is to spend time sitting with the patient and any available family members to map out a good-quality drawing of the pedigree. As much relevant clinical information as possible should be included, even if not immediately of apparent relevance. For example, a grandchild with autism is noteworthy where fragile X tremor ataxia syndrome fits the phenotype. A strong family history of epilepsy, cataracts, or diabetes may favor a mitochondrial cytopathy and a diagnosis of "multiple sclerosis" in older generations before the ready availability of magnetic resonance imaging (MRI) was not always accurate. A well-drawn family tree will be a good point of reference for all future consultations.

PATTERNS OF INHERITANCE

Although when teaching students, we tend to place an emphasis on interpretation of inheritance patterns to guide a search for candidate genes, this is not always helpful in practice. It is certainly useful where there is a clear autosomal dominant pattern of inheritance, guiding testing toward the large family of dominant spinocerebellar ataxias (SCAs). Where parents are unaffected and two or more siblings are affected, particularly if onset is early, a recessive ataxia may be more likely. The conundrum over whether a parent was affected or not is a common problem for geneticists and clinicians when the parent is deceased. Nonpaternity, nonpenetrance in a parent, and death of a parent at an age before onset of ataxia or inaccuracy ("Dad was crippled with arthritis") are all well-known pitfalls in the interpretation of family trees. Repeat questioning and multiple informants will improve yield and accuracy. Sporadic, or more accurately termed "apparently sporadic," cases may of course be truly sporadic but can equally represent a dominant familial ataxia for all the reasons given previously or equally the only affected member of a sibship with a recessive ataxia.

Of course, if clinical details provide compelling support for a specific inherited ataxia, this should be excluded first. For example, a slowly progressive ataxia with teenage onset, areflexia in the lower limbs, scoliosis, and apparently recessive inheritance will always be Friedreich's ataxia until proven otherwise (Fig. 15.1). A dominantly inherited ataxia with dystonia, neuropathy, pyramidal features, and ophthalmoparesis should similarly trigger testing for Machado–Joseph disease (spinocerebellar ataxia type 3 or SCA3). Where there are no distinctive clinical features, most local geneticists will recommend initial testing for the most common genetic ataxic syndromes as a starting point. In some hospitals a precursor of latter-day ataxia panels will exist and include these more common syndromes. In Europe, such panels will typically include testing for triple-repeat expansions associated with Friedreich's ataxia (recessive) and the most common SCAs—SCA1, -2, -3, -6, -7—and occasionally SCA17. Even where the clinical picture does not fit, testing is

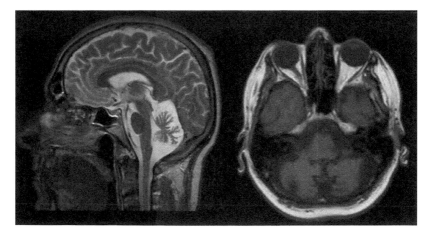

FIGURE 15.1 Cerebellar atrophy in autosomal recessive ataxia due to anoctamin 10 (ANO10) mutations.

typically done regardless because it is relatively cheap using polymerase chain reaction techniques and some laboratories will require it before performing next-generation sequencing, which does not capture these triple-repeat disorders in its current form.

WHERE TO NEXT?

Imaging in familial cerebellar syndromes is typically unhelpful, generally demonstrating nonspecific cerebellar atrophy. Some rare hereditary ataxias have characteristic MRI features that will support direct genetic testing of a specific gene, such as autosomal recessive spastic ataxia of Charlevoix–Saguenay (ARSACS) (Fig. 15.2). A normal-appearing cerebellum can be supportive of Friedreich's ataxia. Until approximately 5 years ago, a negative result on the first initial genetic screen, and an absence of new information or an imaging clue to prompt targeting of an alternative, would commonly have meant an end to diagnostic testing and a diagnosis of an "idiopathic ataxia." An absence of a genetic diagnosis deprives the patient of an explanation for his or her disability, meaningful genetic counseling is not available to families, and the cohorting of homogeneous patient groups for clinical trials is far more difficult. Furthermore, the identification of new genes can assist with the process of unraveling the pathophysiology of individual ataxic syndromes with a view to developing therapies.

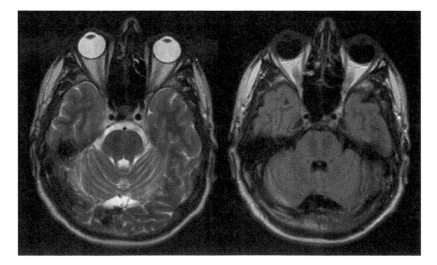

FIGURE 15.2 Linear hypointensities in the pons in autosomal recessive spastic ataxia of Charlevoix–Saguenay (ARSACS).

BACK TO THIS CASE

In this family there is a clear history of ataxia in a sister. If funding was available for further genetic testing, the traditional approach would be to select individual candidate genes for analysis by Sanger sequencing based on the available clinical information. For pure cerebellar ataxias or for spastic ataxias with no distinguishing features otherwise, this exercise is often of low yield and economically inefficient. Frustration can grow for both clinician and patient as successive candidate SCA genes fail to reveal a pathogenic abnormality. The more common recessive ataxias after Friedreich's ataxia, such as ataxia with oculomotor apraxia type 1 and 2 (AOA-1 and AOA-2) and ataxia telangiectasisa, are often checked by virtue of relative familiarity with the phenotype with respect to other recessive syndromes and commercial availability, often without the support of what should be a recognizable phenotype. Further genetic testing of other rare and less recognized recessive syndromes by Sanger sequencing has typically been limited by expense and access.

On a commercially available ataxia panel, this patient was found to have homozygous mutations in the anoctamin 10 gene (*ANO10*), which are associated with recessive ataxic syndromes in the literature. The specific syndrome is an adult-onset autosomal recessive spastic ataxia without neuropathy. As in most non-Friedreich's cerebellar syndromes, cerebellar atrophy is prominent and progressive over time (Fig. 15.3).

THE NEXT-GENERATION SEQUENCING APPROACH

In recent years, there has been a rapid expansion in the availability and success of next-generation sequencing (NGS) techniques in the diagnosis of neurological disease. NGS is a method of sequencing large numbers of genes in a short amount of time at a cost similar to that of sequencing individual genes using Sanger sequencing. The appropriate "panel" of genes can be chosen to fit the broad phenotype (i.e., ataxia, parkinsonism, or hereditary spastic paraparesis). It is important to be aware of overlap between phenotypes where the spastic ataxias are concerned. Mutations in paraplegin (SPG7) have been identified as a potentially common cause of a spastic ataxia, despite being classified among the hereditary spastic paraplegias. Ataxic syndromes lend themselves to this approach due to the difficulty in identifying a gene to check in a cerebellar syndrome with no distinguishing characteristics other than a nonspecific axonal neuropathy or lower limb spasticity. The number of genes covered by commercially available panels continues to expand as new genes are identified. This

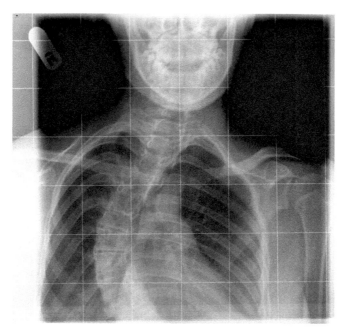

FIGURE 15.3 Thoracic kyphoscoliosis in Friedreich's ataxia.

approach has been shown to achieve a genetic diagnosis in more than 50% of patients who have no genetic diagnosis despite a strong clinical suspicion of a heritable ataxic syndrome.

WHAT DO YOU DO IF THE ATAXIA PANEL IDENTIFIES A VARIANT OF UNCERTAIN SIGNIFICANCE OR NO ABNORMALITY AT ALL?

An inevitable consequence of sequencing a large number of base pairs is the identification of variants, of which each person carries tens of thousands. Where a variant has been reported to be associated with disease in the literature, it is has been traditionally called a mutation and the term polymorphism is often used when a variant is believed to be benign. It is now preferred that all base pair alterations are called variants and that the pathogenicity of these variants is classified on a scale from pathogenic to benign. It is the variants of "unknown significance" that cause difficulty and require further interpretation. Commercial laboratories will search a number of international databases to look for reported disease associations in other populations. In silico or computational modeling of the consequence of any variant at a nucleotide or base pair level can also help inform pathogenicity. Where possible, assessment of other family members can be informative, particularly when there are other affected family members, to determine if the variant segregates with disease in the family.

Where no potentially pathogenic abnormality can be found, whole exome sequencing (WES) is increasingly becoming the next step in the diagnostic algorithm where there is a sufficiently strong case to be made for a genetic disorder. Whereas a panel relies on the core phenotypic feature to choose the selection of the appropriate phenotype (i.e., ataxia vs. parkinsonism), WES provides unselected analysis of the entire coding region of the genome. Even with this, there is a potential to miss intronic disorders and triple-repeat disorders. As technology improves to provide for cheaper and more rapid results, the horizon broadens, with whole genome sequencing encompassing triple-repeat and mitochondrial disorders the ultimate end point. The challenge in interpreting variants will multiply as this happens, although so too will our ability to give patients and families information that until recently they have had little expectation of receiving.

KEY POINTS TO REMEMBER

- When considering a familial ataxic syndrome, always begin with and record a detailed family tree derived from as many informants as possible.
- It is likely that a significant subset of patients attending with what appears to be a sporadic ataxic syndrome are actually the only family member manifesting a recessive ataxic syndrome; genetic testing is equally valid once acquired syndromes have been excluded.
- Our ability to identify a genetic diagnosis in inherited ataxic syndromes has improved significantly since the advent of next-generation sequencing techniques employed in commercially available gene panels.
- Although expensive, the use of gene panels is significantly more cost-effective than gene-by-gene analysis using Sanger sequencing. However, the latter is still in use for confirmation of any abnormality found using the NGS approach.

Further Reading

Keogh MJ, Steele H, Douroudis K, et al. Frequency of rare recessive mutations in unexplained late onset cerebellar ataxia. *J Neurol* 2015 Aug;262(8):1822–1827.

Németh AH, Kwasniewska AC, Lise S, et al. Next generation sequencing for molecular diagnosis of neurological disorders using ataxias as a model. *Brain* 2013 Oct;136(10):3106–3118.

Pfeffer G, Pyle A, Griffin H, et al. SPG7 mutations are a common cause of undiagnosed ataxia. *Neurology* 2015 Mar 17;84(11):1174–1176.

16 Parkinson's Disease or Essential Tremor?

Richard A. Walsh

You are assessing a 63-year-old man who has been referred for consideration of deep-brain stimulation for an essential tremor after his doctor found him unresponsive to propranolol, primidone, and a number of other agents. He reports onset of tremor in his late 50s, with a slow evolution of imbalance during the past 3 years, which his neurologist had attributed to cerebellar pathology in essential tremor. He derives no benefit from ingestion of alcohol. There is no family history of tremor. His daughter has a son with autism. On examination he has mild hypomimia. There is a postural and action tremor that is predominantly flexion–extension at the wrist and is terminal worsening. There is also head involvement, which is "yes–yes" in nature. There is no vocal involvement. On lower limb examination there is mild to moderate heel–shin dysmetria and a symmetrical reduction in sensation to vibration, present only at the costal margin. Ankle jerks are absent. Gait assessment reveals a mild to moderate ataxia with need of a stick for stability and an inability to heel–toe walk.

What do you do now?

FRAGILE X-ASSOCIATED TREMOR ATAXIA SYNDROME

As in every situation in which you receive a referral for specialist management of a specific syndrome, your first task is to satisfy yourself as to the accuracy of the original diagnosis. Perpetuation of an earlier misdiagnosis is a disservice to both the patient and the referring physician. In this case, the man referred has not unreasonably been given a diagnosis of essential tremor, presumably based on the tremor phenomenology and the fact that essential tremor is by far the most common form of "isolated" tremor disorder. The presence of cognitive features and gait ataxia, however, should raise suspicion of an alternative diagnosis. It is important to recognize that cognitive impairment and gait disturbance are now well-reported features of essential tremor, but they are typically seen in older patients in whom there may be coexisting pathologies.

Mild neuropathic features on examination are not in keeping with essential tremor, although peripheral neuropathy can also be an independent phenomenon in an older patient, unrelated to the presenting complaint. Perhaps of most benefit when attempting to resolve the differential diagnosis here is the family history of autism or what has been called "autism." Given the prevalence of the carrier status, the fragile X-associated tremor ataxia syndrome (FXTAS) should be considered in any patient with one or more of the core clinical features of tremor, ataxia, and mild cognitive impairment. A family history of a male grandchild or nephew born to a daughter or niece should heighten this suspicion.

PATHOPHYSIOLOGY

FXTAS is a neurodegenerative disorder associated with a CGG triple-repeat premutation in a noncoding segment of the fragile X mental retardation 1 (*FMR1*) gene, first described in 2001. The normal *FMR1* gene CGG repeat length is less than 40, with repeat lengths of greater than 200 (or a full mutation) being associated with fragile X, a related neurodevelopmental disorder presenting in childhood characterized by intellectual disability and typical facial features. Triple-repeat segments between 55 and 200 repeats, or premutations, are associated with a risk of developing FXTAS. Unlike in fragile X syndrome, in which a full mutation gives rise to a loss of FMR1 protein synthesis, a premutation results in toxic gain of function with elevated intracellular *FMR1* mRNA and subsequent neurodegeneration. There is a gray zone (45–54 repeats) for which there is evidence for increased intracellular FMR1 mRNA and case reports of individuals with clinical features in keeping with FXTAS. The pathological substrate in FXTAS is widespread glial and neuronal eosinophilic inclusions that are ubiquitin positive and tau and synuclein negative. These inclusions do not contain *FMR1* mRNA.

As with all X-linked disorders, female carriers are protected by the presence of a second X chromosome. Similarly, male children of men who are carriers of a premutation or full mutation will not be at risk because a father's X chromosome is passed on to female offspring who will become obligatory carriers. Skewed lyonization is believed to be responsible for rendering some female carriers symptomatic. Penetrance in female premutation carriers older than age 50 years is estimated to be approximately 15%, compared to 40% among male carriers of the same age group, with evidence of increased penetrance with advancing years.

CLINICAL MANIFESTATIONS

Mean age of onset is in the seventh decade, with only rare cases presenting after age 50 years. Tremor, ataxia, cognitive impairment, and sensorimotor neuropathy are the most common clinical features of FXTAS. The tremor is typically an action tremor but can be seen at rest in one-third of patients. As in the case of the patient presented here, the tremor can look identical to essential tremor, and it is likely that many neurologists have made this misdiagnosis on at least one occasion. An increasing number of nonmotor symptoms are being recognized as the phenotype expands, with case recognition being supported by the diagnosis of fragile X syndrome in young male relatives (Box 16.1).

In women permutation carriers, FXTAS can present with a phenotype indistinguishable from that of their male counterparts; however, a milder phenotype with some additional features is more common. Premature ovarian failure (<40 years of age) is seen in 20%; fibromyalgia-type symptoms are more common than in the general population; and there appears to be a higher prevalence of hypothyroidism and hypertension, which should be screened for in males and females. White matter disease and atrophy on magnetic resonance imaging (MRI) are less common in women and in keeping with this dementia appear to be less common in female permutation carriers.

INVESTIGATION

MRI of brain should be considered in any patient being treated for essential tremor who fails to respond to the most effective oral therapies, such as

Motor

> Ataxia
> Tremor
> Parkinsonism
> Focal dystonia
> Stimulus-sensitive myoclonus
> Myopathy

Nonmotor

> Peripheral neuropathy (large > small fiber)
> Autonomic neuropathy
> Premature ovarian failure
> Impaired olfaction

Neuropsychiatric and cognitive

> Anxiety/depression
> Cognitive or behavioral change
> Frontal dysexecutive and/or amnestic MCI
> Dementia

Neurodevelopmental

> Autism spectrum disorder
> Attention deficit hyperactivity disorder
> Seizure diathesis

propranolol and primidone, and who has additional atypical features. Any patient with an undiagnosed cerebellar syndrome or atypical parkinsonism who has a grandson or nephew with an intellectual disability should also be considered for imaging. A patient presenting with a multiple system atrophy-like syndrome with onset after age 65 years may also warrant an MRI of brain, although most patients with this presentation will already have had this performed.

No imaging finding in FXTAS is pathognomonic for the condition; however, in the right clinical context (for criteria, see Table 16.1), the more specific imaging findings of hyperintensity of the middle cerebellar peduncle (Fig. 16.1) or splenium of the corpus callosum should prompt genetic testing. Importantly, more than one-third of patients with FXTAS will have none of the imaging

TABLE 16.1 Revised Criteria for Diagnosis of FXTAS Where Gray Zone Mutation, Permutation, or Full Mutation of the _FMR1_ Gene Is Identified

FXTAS Category	Exam and Degree
Definite	Clinical
One major clinical and	_Major_—Cerebellar ataxia
One major radiological	_Major_—Action tremor
or	_Minor_—Autonomic dysfunction
Pathological confirmation	_Minor_—Moderate to severe short-term memory deficit
	Minor—Executive dysfunction
	Minor—Neuropathy
Probable	
Two major clinical	Radiological
or	_Major_—Middle cerebellar peduncle hyperintensities
Two minor clinical and	_Major_—Hyperintensity of the corpus callosum splenium
one major radiological	_Minor_—Subcortical white matter intensities
	Minor—Moderate to severe generalized atrophy
Possible	
One major clinical and	Pathological
one radiological minor	Typical pathological findings of FXTAS

Source: Adapted with permission from Hall DA, Birch RC, Anheim M, et al. Emerging topics in FXTAS. _J Neurodev Disord_ 2014;6(1):31.

characteristics described, and genetic testing for the CGG expansion is the only other diagnostic option.

PRACTICAL CONSIDERATIONS IN FXTAS

As with all neurodegenerative disorders, currently there is no specific therapy available to target progression of disability in FXTAS. Most patients will benefit from involvement with the full multidisciplinary team to allow assessment at

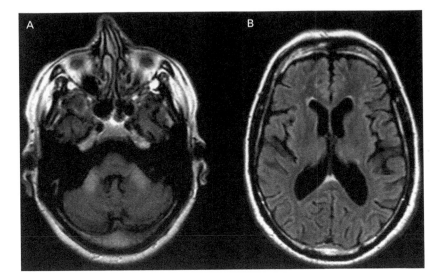

FIGURE 16.1 (A) Bilateral middle cerebellar peduncle hyperintensities in a patient with FXTAS. (B) Hyperintensity of the splenium of the corpus callosum in the same patient.

home for the necessary adaptations. Formal neuropsychological assessment is an important element of this given the prominent cognitive and neuropsychiatric features. Caregiver burden among carers of patients with FXTAS can be considerable for the same reason, and with progression of disability and dementia in some cases respite admissions and assistance from a social worker are valuable. Some patients with prominent behavioral change, depression, or anxiety will also benefit from a formal psychiatry review.

From a symptomatic perspective, there are no randomized controlled trials to guide physicians in their choice of antitremor agent. Some patients may obtain some relief from agents used in essential tremor, and many patients will have been tried on these prior to your assessment. FXTAS, like any postural tremor, may benefit from beta-blockers, although caution is required due to the potential coexistence of orthostatic hypotension secondary to comorbid autonomic neuropathy. Primidone and topiramate may also be considered. There are case reports of benefit from deep-brain stimulation, although, as in Parkinson's disease, postural instability and cognitive impairment will continue to deteriorate and even worsen despite a tremor response.

As with any genetic condition, genetic counseling should be made available to any interested family members, particularly daughters or affected patients who are obligate carriers due to considerations with regard to pregnancy and the risk of having a child with a full mutation (>200 CGG repeats) associated with fragile X syndrome.

- FXTAS is an X-linked disorder manifesting in carriers of a premutation in the *FMR1* gene. The carrier prevalence is high, being found in approximately 1 in 250 females and 1 in 450 males, with estimates varying considerably in different regions and according to methods of case ascertainment.
- Fragile X tremor ataxia syndrome can look identical to essential tremor in terms of its phenomenology where the ataxic component is not prominent. Careful assessment should be performed for associated features, including cognitive impairment, autonomic features, and peripheral neuropathy.
- MRI of brain can be particularly informative if revealing the classic bilateral hyperintensity of the middle cerebellar peduncles and splenium of the corpus callosum on T2-weighted MRI sequences, which although not pathognomonic are supportive of FXTAS in the right clinical context.
- Obtaining a detailed family history remains a key part of any patient history, not just with respect to "any neurological diseases" but specifically looking for nieces, nephews, and grandchildren with learning disabilities or developmental delay that may not be attributed to neurological disease.

Further Reading

Eye PG, Hawley JS. Pearls & Oy-sters: Fragile X tremor/ataxia syndrome: A diagnostic dilemma. *Neurology* 2015 Feb 17;84(7):e43–e45.

Greco CM, Hagerman RJ, Tassone F, et al. Neuronal intranuclear inclusions in a new cerebellar tremor/ataxia syndrome among fragile X carriers. *Brain* 2002 Aug;125(Pt 8):1760–1771.

Hall DA, Birch RC, Anheim M, et al. Emerging topics in FXTAS. *J Neurodev Disord* 2014;6(1):31.

Hagerman R, Hagerman P. Advances in clinical and molecular understanding of the FMR1 premutation and fragile X-associated tremor/ataxia syndrome. *Lancet Neurol* 2013 Aug;12(8):786–798.

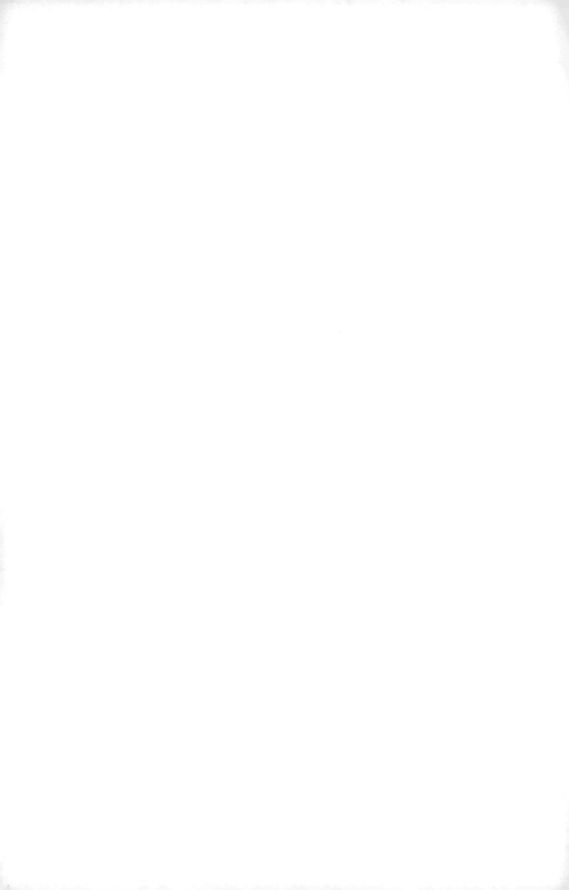

PART IV

Dystonia

17 Seizures and Shakes

Susan H. Fox

An 18-year-old male is referred with two generalized seizures in the past 6 months and paroxysmal shaking in his legs. He was seen by a local neurologist who diagnosed primary generalized epilepsy and prescribed sodium valproate. His parents are worried because he has also become more withdrawn and ambivalent and they think he is depressed. There is a family history of depression and suicide. He works part-time at a local store and did well at school. There are no significant prior medical issues, and he denies any illicit drug use.

On examination he is alert and orientated but distracted and not engaging in conversation. Speech and language are normal. He has reduced facial expression and some intermittent grimacing in his lower face. He has a mild postural and kinetic tremor on outstretched hands. He has dystonic posturing in his hands and in turning of the right foot, which increases when performing foot-tapping movements. On walking he has a "bouncy," stiff-legged broad-based gait.

What do you do now?

WILSON'S DISEASE

Examine the Eyes

The combination of a mixed movement disorder, tremor, dystonia, and possible ataxic gait with neuropsychiatric symptoms in a young person should always make you think of Wilson's disease (Table 17.1). In clinic, check for Kayser–Fleisher (KF) rings (golden-brown pigmentation around the cornea starting in

TABLE 17.1 Differential Diagnosis of Tremor with Dystonia/Parkinsonism in a Young Person

Disorders	Causes—Genetic Mutation
Drug-induced	Dopamine D2 receptor antagonists (e.g., antipsychotics)
	Illicit drugs (e.g., toluene sniffing); manganese toxicity (methcathinone abuse from over-the-counter cold remedies containing ephedrine or pseudoephedrine)
Wilson's disease	>500 mutations in the gene *ATP7B* (http://www.wilsondisease.med.ualberta.ca/database.asp)
Huntington's disease	Juvenile variant of HD due to large expansion, >60 CAG repeats in HD gene
Huntington's disease-like disorders	HDL-1, *PRNP*; HDL2, *JPH3*; HDL-4, *TBP1*
	C9orf72 expansion is most common cause of HD-like disorder
Genetic parkinsonism	Common: PARK2, *parkin*; PARK8, *LRRK2*; PARK6, *pink-1*; PARK7, *DJ1*
	Rare: PARK1, *SNCA*; PARK9 (Kufor–Rakeb disease), *ATP13A2*; PARK15, *FBOX7*; PARK17, *VP35*; PARK19, *DNAJC6*; PARK20, *SYNJ1*
Genetic dystonias	Dopa-responsive dystonia: DYT5, *GCH1, TH, SPR*
	Other genetic dystonias: DYT3, *TAF1*; DYT12, *ATP1A3*
Neuronal brain iron accumulation disorders	Pantothenate kinase-associated neurodegeneration (PKAN), *PANK2*
	Phospholipase A$_2$-associated neurodegeneration (PLAN), *PLA2G6*
	Mitochondrial membrane-associated neurodegeneration (MPAN), *C19orf12*
	Beta-propeller-associated neurodegeneration (BPAN), *WDR45*
Metabolic	Renal/liver failure

superior pole and spreading to lower pole) using an ophthalmoscope. However, referral for slit-lamp examination is required for confirmation because KF rings may be difficult to see in subjects with brown eyes. KF rings are diagnostic of neurological Wilson's disease (false positives can occur in primary biliary cirrhosis and false negative in very early onset Wilson's disease).

What Further Tests Do You Organize?

Send serum for liver function tests (liver disease is common in Wilson's disease, ranging from acute hepatitis, chronic active hepatitis to cirrhosis). Check renal and hematological function with a renal profile and full blood count, respectively. The gold standard diagnostic test is a liver biopsy that shows increased copper content: 200–250 µg/g copper (normal, 20–50 µg). Ultrastructural changes of enlarged vacuoles and mitochondrial abnormalities in the absence of cholestasis are pathognomonic. Copper studies including 24-hour urinary copper excretion (using a copper-free collecting container) are sent before consideration of the more invasive liver biopsy. An abnormal result is increased copper excretion in excess of 100 µg (or >1.57 µmol/24 hours); the value should be at least twice the normal level to be diagnostic. Serum ceruloplasmin is low in Wilson's disease, <0.2 g/liter (normal, >0.3 g/liter). The key is not to overinterpret borderline or marginally altered results that are common and may be false positives (due to other liver disease or a heterozygote carrier state). In such cases, repeat the tests. Brain magnetic resonance imaging (MRI) is extremely useful to confirm neurological Wilson's disease and is invariably abnormal with copper deposition in the basal ganglia causing high signal changes on T2 in basal ganglia, brainstem, and cortex. White matter changes can also occur and may indicate a poor prognosis. Genetic testing for the *ATP7B* gene will not 100% exclude the diagnosis due to the large number of mutations (>600) reported.

BACK TO THE CASE

The 24-hour urinary copper excretion was 110 µg/24 hours, the ceruloplasmin was low (0.1 g/liter), and ophthalmology examination using slit lamp demonstrated the presence of KF rings. A brain MRI also showed the classic "face of the giant panda" on T2 signal on midbrain cuts. This confirmed the diagnosis of Wilson's disease. However, you are still unsure about the epilepsy and whether to continue with the anti-convulsant. The combination of a movement disorder with epilepsy is unusual but does occur (Table 17.2). The cause of the seizures was thought to be due to Wilson's disease. The patient was started on trientine and slowly started to improve. After 18 months, he was switched to

TABLE 17.2 **Movement Disorders Associated with Epileptic Seizures (Excluding Myoclonic Syndromes)**

Condition	Phenomenology of Movement Disorders	Seizure Disorder
Huntington's disease and Huntington's disease-like disorders	Chorea, later parkinsonism and dystonia; tics	Generalized tonic–clonic seizures; tonic, staring spells
Neuroacanthocytosis	Choreoathetosis; tics; parkinsonism	Focal
Neuronal brain iron accumulation disorders	dystonia, parkinsonism, choreoathetosis	Generalized
Primary familial brain calcification	Parkinsonism; tremor	Generalized tonic–clonic seizures
Wilson's disease	Dystonia; tremor; parkinsonism	Generalized tonic–clonic seizures
Paroxysmal kinesogenic dyskinesia (PRRT2) Exercise-induced dyskinesia (GLUT-1)	Kinesiogenic or exercise-induced chorea/dystonia	Benign familial infantile seizures; idiopathic generalized epilepsy
Autoimmune encephalitis (e.g., due to NMDA receptor antibody)	Chorea	Generalized tonic–clonic seizures
Rett's syndrome	Stereotypies	Tonic, generalized clonic, partial, absence

zinc monotherapy; he continued to have a slow improvement during the course of 2½ years. He had no further seizures, and sodium valproate was discontinued after 3 months.

WILSON'S DISEASE AND EPILEPSY

Epileptic seizures are described in Wilsons' disease and can occur in up to 10% of cases. The timing of seizures is usually in the early stages of the disease, and approximately 20% occur before other symptoms, approximately 50% occur concurrently with other symptoms of Wilson's disease, and approximately 30% occur after treatment is started and can be associated with neurological worsening with de-coppering agents. All types of seizures have been described, but generalized tonic–clonic seizures are most common. There may be electroencephalographic correlates of seizure activity. The prognosis is generally good, with approximately three-fourths becoming seizure-free. A possible link between white matter changes on MRI and intractable seizures, and also poor clinical motor and neurological outcomes, has been suggested.

KEY POINTS TO REMEMBER

- Wilson's disease is a disorder that should not be missed, and any patient presenting with a movement disorder before the age of 50 years should have serum and urinary copper checked.
- Unusual "funny" tremors, psychiatric issues, and dystonia in a young person are clinical indicators to investigate for Wilson's disease.
- Epilepsy can occur in up to 10% of patients with Wilson's disease and may respond to copper chelation therapy.
- Treatment needs to be monitored by a neurologist and liver clinic, and patients need to be advised that improvement will take 1 or 2 years.

Further Reading

Aggarwal A, Bhatt M. The pragmatic treatment of Wilson's disease. *Mov Disord Clin Pract* 2014;1:14–23.

Pfeiffer RF. Wilson's disease. *AAN Continuum* 2016; in press.

Prashanth LK, Sinha S, Taly AB, et al. Spectrum of epilepsy in Wilson's disease with electroencephalographic, MR imaging and pathological correlates. *J Neurol Sci* 2010;291(1–2):44–51.

18 A Tremor with an Abnormal Posture

Robertus M. A. de Bie and
Susanne E. M. Ten Holter

You see a 70-year-old male with a tremor in both hands since 8 years of age. Initially, the tremor started in his left hand and was only present during action. The tremor has progressed: The right arm became involved; the amplitude of the tremor increased; and although it is still more prominent during action, it is now also present when the arms rest. He experiences difficulties with daily activities such as dressing, eating, or making repairs around the house. He did not notice tremor in other body parts. Several drugs have been tried but were not helpful. On examination, he has a mild rest tremor of his left hand and a severe postural and intention tremor in both hands. The tremor is of large amplitude and has a moderate frequency. There is no proximal tremor in the arms and no tremor of the head. However, there is asymmetry of the shoulders, the left shoulder appears elevated, and intermittently the patient displays a subtle rotation of the head with the chin to the left.

What do you do now?

DYSTONIC TREMOR

Differential Diagnosis

When dealing with a patient with tremor, the first step is to define the tremor type using the patient history and clinical assessment. Important features are the location of the tremor (i.e., limb, head, voice, trunk, and symmetry); the frequency of the tremor; and whether the tremor occurs when the body part is at rest, in action, or in posture, during an intentional movement, or a combination of these. A frequency of less than 4 Hz is considered a low frequency, 4–7 Hz is considered a medium frequency, and greater than 7 Hz is considered a high frequency. In this case the initial presentation appeared to meet the criteria for essential tremor. For essential tremor, however, other neurological features should be absent. The elevated shoulder and the rotation of the head indicate dystonia. Therefore, this tremor is a tremor associated with dystonia.

Dystonia and Tremor Classification

Dystonia is an involuntary sustained muscular contraction resulting in twisting movements or abnormal postures. Where a patient has dystonia and tremor, the classification presented here may be used.

The first type is dystonic tremor (DT), in which a postural and/or kinetic tremor is present in a body region affected by the dystonia—for example, cervical dystonia with a head tremor. The second type is tremor associated with dystonia (TAD or TAWD). In these patients, the tremor is present in other body parts besides those with the dystonia. The last type is the dystonia–gene associated tremor. This tremor is an isolated symptom in a patient with a known dystonia gene mutation, and there is often a positive family history for dystonia. When a patient presents with tremor, the dystonia may be already known. However, the dystonia may also be very subtle; therefore, attention should be paid to clues that indicate dystonia while examining the patient. If a patient has both dystonia and tremor, the symptoms are classified as a dystonic tremor syndrome, even if the dystonia is not the most prominent feature. Exceptions to this rule are the cases in which the tremor and dystonia occur as part of another known disorder, such as Parkinson's disease. Although different presentations of these tremor types (DT, TAWD, and dystonia gene-associated tremor) are recognized, there is speculation in the literature that these are different expressions of the same pathology.

Clinical Features

Tremor can occur in every type of dystonia. Tremor of the head or a limb is seen most often, but the tremor can occur in any other body part. There is not a general distribution or characteristic. Frequently, the tremor is postural and kinetic, but it can also appear during rest. When the characteristics of the tremor do not fit a specific type of tremor (e.g., rest and postural tremor in Parkinson's disease and a predominantly high-frequency postural tremor as in physiological tremor) or changes over time, a dystonic tremor type should be considered. Frequency and amplitude can be irregular, and the tremor can vary during different postures and motor tasks. It can, for example, worsen when moving away from the direction of the dystonia or diminish after sensory stimuli (also referred to as antagonistic gestures or sensory tricks) or when the favorable position for the dystonia is taken. These symptoms are clues for a dystonic tremor type. A primary head tremor without other symptoms is uncommon for an essential tremor and is suspected to be a dystonic tremor as well.

When observing a patient with tremor, it is important to be alert for possible dystonia. Therefore, it is essential to know what features to expect. The more common focal dystonia types are as follows:

- Cervical dystonia: This can include various combinations of rotation, lateroflexion, ante- or retrocollis, or shoulder elevation.
- Focal dystonia, most often of a hand and in adult patients typically task specific: Examples are writer's cramp and musician's cramp. Patients experience difficulty performing these specific tasks due to the dystonia. Sometimes the dystonia is evident when asking to perform the specific task with the other hand. This can be as subtle as posturing of the thumb. The extension of the thumb can resemble a "thumbs up" and has been referred to as the "Fonzarelli" sign because of the characteristic gesture of "Arthur Fonzarelli" in the television series *Happy Days*. An extension of the big toe can also be seen.
- Blepharospasm due to dystonia of the orbicularis oculi muscles resulting in squeezing of the eyes.
- Oromandibular dystonia occurring mainly in the jaw with opening or closing of the jaw, which can worsen during talking and eating.
- Laryngeal dystonia, also referred to as vocal dystonia or spasmodic dysphonia: This is a task-specific dystonia affecting the voice and resulting in a pinched voice (adductor dysphonia) or a large amount of air escaping during speech (abductor dysphonia). A voice tremor may occur.

Diagnosis

The underlying pathophysiology of tremor that accompanies dystonia is not precisely known. The tremor is probably caused by a similar basal ganglia lesion or "network impairment" that underlies the dystonia. The diagnosis of dystonic tremor is a clinical diagnosis just like the diagnosis of essential tremor and can be very challenging, especially because the presentation can be very diverse. However, regardless of the tremor features, if dystonia is present and there is no other known disease, the tremor is classified as dystonic tremor syndrome (either a dystonic tremor or a tremor associated with dystonia). Common pitfalls are the intermittent dystonia occurring only during voluntary movements or the very subtle and difficult to recognize dystonia, which makes it difficult to distinguish the dystonic tremor from essential tremor. No diagnostic test is available to distinguish a dystonic tremor from an essential tremor. Because dystonic tremors may appear in rest, they can mimic parkinsonian tremor. In this case, a dopamine transporter scan can give clarity because reduced presynaptic binding of the ligand as seen in, for example, Parkinson's disease is not expected in dystonic tremor.

Treatment

Treatment tends to be difficult because there is often little effect of medication. There are no randomized controlled trials, and in most studies the different types of dystonic tremor syndromes are not acknowledged. Anticholinergic drugs, mostly trihexiphenidyl up to 4–10 mg per day, are regularly tried. Tremor amplitude may be reduced with variable efficacy. Often treatment regimens for essential tremor are tried; a few reports of beta-blocking agents and primidone are published, which show variable efficacy. Benzodiazepines (primarily clonazepam) have also been mentioned in the literature with a variable effect. Interestingly, total disappearance of the tremor was seen in a small number of patients in one series; the authors referred to this tremor as "clonazepam sensitive dystonic tremor." In dopamine responsive dystonia, an effect was seen on the dystonia as well as on the associated tremor following treatment with levodopa. Intramuscular botulinum toxin injection, preventing acetylcholine release in the neuromuscular junction and inducing a chemical denervation of the muscle, seems to have better success than oral drugs. It can be of use in the treatment of tremor in the dystonic segment, with the best results for head tremor. Tremor in extremities or tremor in a nondystonic segment do not benefit as satisfactorily from botulinum toxin. Transcutaneous electrical nerve stimulation has shown no efficacy. When dealing with a medically refractory tremor that causes disability, functional neurosurgery can be considered. Currently, in most surgical centers performing deep-brain stimulation (DBS), the globus pallidus is targeted for dystonia. For essential tremor, the thalamic ventral intermediate nucleus (VIM) is the DBS target of choice. Although the pathophysiology of dystonic tremor is expected to be different from that of essential tremor, the best tremor reduction seems to be accomplished when targeting the VIM. DBS targeting the VIM, however, may have only a minimal effect on dystonia. Therefore, when the dystonia is also prominent, the globus pallidus should be the primary target. In exceptional cases, both the globus pallidus and VIM are targeted.

Our patient is severely disabled due to the dystonic tremor, and an adequate medical treatment has already been tried. Therefore, DBS should be considered. Because his most prominent feature is the tremor and not the dystonia, we would opt for targeting the VIM.

KEY POINTS TO REMEMBER

- A tremor in the presence of a dystonia is a dystonic tremor syndrome, regardless of the clinical features.
- Alertness for dystonia when analyzing a patient with tremor is essential to differentiate the dystonic tremor from other tremor syndromes.
- Botulinum toxin injections or, in refractory cases, DBS are treatment options for dystonic tremor syndromes.

Further Reading

Albanese A, Bhatia K, Bressman SB, et al. Phenomenology and classification of dystonia: A consensus update. *Mov Disord* 2013;28:863–873.

Fasano A, Bove F, Lang AE. The treatment of dystonic tremor: A systematic review. *J Neurol Neurosurg Psychiatry* 2014;85:759–769.

Hedera P, Phibbs FT, Dolhun R, et al. Surgical targets for dystonic tremor: Considerations between the globus pallidus and ventral intermediate thalamic nucleus. *Parkinsonism Relat Disord* 2013;19:684–6.

Schneider SA, Edwards MJ, Mir P, et al. Patients with adult-onset dystonic tremor resembling parkinsonian tremor have scans without evidence of dopaminergic deficit (SWEDDs). *Mov Disord* 2007;22:2210–2215.

19 Advanced Treatment for Dystonia

Robertus M. A. de Bie and
Susanne E. M. Ten Holter

For 10 years, you have been treating a 55-year-old female schoolteacher with cervical dystonia. In the beginning there was a relatively good effect of treatment with intramuscular botulinum toxin injections, but in the past 4 years, despite revised schemes, the effect has waned. You do not expect any benefit from more adjustments of the regimen, and you considered the possibility of botulinum toxin resistance. However, this appeared not to be the case. Systemic treatment using trihexyphenidyl and diazepam did not improve the cervical dystonia, and increasing the dose was not tolerated because of side effects. Currently, she has a rotation of more than 30 degrees to the right, an elevation of the right shoulder, a slight retroflexion, and an almost continuous head tremor. Voluntary neck movements are limited, and the patient experiences pain in the neck. She is severely limited in her work. She does not feel fit to drive, and although she used to be active in tennis and yoga, she had to stop both due to the cervical dystonia.

What do you do now?

SELECTING CANDIDATES FOR DEEP BRAIN STIMULATION IN DYSTONIA

In this case the cervical dystonia is severe, has a considerable impact in daily life, and interferes with the patient's job abilities. Medical treatment in the form of chemical denervation with botulinum toxin injections and medication has been tried adequately but in the end with an unsatisfactory result. The next step to consider is bilateral deep brain stimulation (DBS) of the internal part of the globus pallidus (GPi).

Indication for Deep Brain Stimulation

Several criteria should be met before considering a referral for DBS. First, it is very important that there is a correct diagnosis of dystonia and some understanding of the etiology. Treatable causes of dystonia should be explored. Examples of treatable forms are dystonia due to a metabolic disorder or levodopa-responsive dystonia. The etiology of the dystonia can help to predict the efficacy of treatment with DBS. To justify an invasive treatment such as DBS, there has to be a considerable disability due to the disease. However, this should be interpreted broadly; for example, disability could be the motor restrictions but also the psychosocial limitations. It is important to consider whether the dystonia is the predominant source of disability or if there are other factors influencing the quality of life in a negative way. Other indicated treatments should have been tried adequately. In the case of generalized dystonia, systemic treatment is the first choice. Anticholinergic drugs (trihexyphenidyl), a gamma-aminobutyric acid agonist (baclofen), and the benzodiazepines clozapine and tetrabenazine are different treatment options. In secondary dystonia, intrathecal baclofen should be considered. Titrating systemic medication is often limited by side effects. For focal or segmental dystonia, the first choice is intramuscular injections with botulinum toxin. If there is not enough benefit, revision of the botulinum toxin treatment scheme should be considered or systemic medication can be added. Contraindications for DBS should be considered as well. Psychiatric comorbidity, especially depression, is a relative contraindication for DBS because the prevalence of anxiety and depressive disorders is higher after DBS and suicide has been reported in patients who had suicidal thoughts before surgery. Other contraindications are an indication for anticoagulant therapy without the possibility of stopping it temporarily or a coagulopathy, the inability to understand the consequences or how to use the DBS devices (e.g., dementia), and another serious illness (e.g., cardiovascular disease and hepatic or renal failure).

Deep Brain Stimulation Workup

If a patient is considered to be candidate for DBS, a screening will be performed in the hospital performing the surgery. This will include blood tests (e.g., coagulation parameters), magnetic resonance imaging (to exclude causes of secondary dystonia and to secure the pathways to reach the DBS targets), and a psychiatric and cognitive evaluation. The findings are then discussed in a multidisciplinary team before granting the operation.

Deep Brain Stimulation Target

For DBS, the best evidence for efficacy in dystonia is for surgeries with placement of the electrodes in the GPi. A few smaller studies implicate a role for stimulation of the subthalamic nucleus. Most often the procedure is performed bilaterally, but in cases in which there is a profound lateralization, unilateral implantation could be considered.

Complications

There are three categories of complications in DBS surgery: perioperative complications, hardware complications, and complications due to stimulation. Perioperative complications can be due to anesthetics or to the implantation itself. A hemorrhage is seen in 3% of patients and in 1% with permanent neurologic impairments. An epileptic fit can occur during implantation or in the weeks following surgery (up to 3% of patients). Hardware complications include infection of the implanted material, often needing to remove the material and implanting it when the infection is treated, migration of the material, and breaking of a lead. These complications are seen more frequently in dystonia compared to other movement disorders (18% vs. 4%), probably because of the force on the leads due to cervical and axial dystonic posturing. This is a potentially dangerous complication because a sudden disconnection may lead to a status dystonicus. Stimulation-related side effects are related to the placement of the leads in the GPi and the surrounding structures (e.g., internal capsule, optic tracts, and thalamus), and dysarthria, muscle cramps, paresthesias, and light flashes can be experienced. Also, bradykinesia, rigidity, or freezing can be a side effect of GPi stimulation. These symptoms occur relatively often, but they mostly disappear after adjusting the settings of the electrode. As mentioned previously, suicide has been reported postoperative. Therefore, a careful psychiatric follow-up is advised.

Results

The effect of DBS can set in gradually, several weeks or even months after placement of the leads, in contrast to DBS for tremor or Parkinson's disease, where an effect may already be seen during surgery. To establish the effect of DBS for dystonia, the Burke–Fahn–Marsden Dystonia Rating Scale (BFMDRS) is used, and the Toronto Western Spasmodic Torticollis Rating Scale (TWSTRS) is used for cervical dystonia. These scales measure the amount of disability. A variety of scales are used to measure quality of life. Because dystonia is a heterogenic disease, general prediction of outcome is very difficult. A new classification for dystonia was introduced in 2013 by the Parkinson's Disease and Movement Disorders Society and categorizes dystonia as inherited, acquired (dystonia due to a known specific cause such as brain injury, infection, or drugs), or idiopathic. The (older) literature, however, uses the previous classification in which the dystonia types were considered primary or secondary dystonia.

In general, patients with inherited or idiopathic dystonia experience a gratifying effect of DBS. The presence of the disease for more than 15 years has a less favorable outcome, probably because of fixed deformities and contractures. Phasic dystonia improves earlier and more than static dystonia, and oromandibular involvement has a less favorable outcome.

Inherited or Idiopathic Dystonia

Primary generalized dystonia is the best-analyzed group and has a good response of 50–60% on the BFMDRS with a stable postoperative follow-up of up to 10 years. The effect is similar for *DYT1*-positive and -negative patients, but patients with a *DYT6* mutation are less likely to benefit. This difference is probably due to a prominent laryngeal and craniocervical involvement and the disappointing response on dystonic-related speech impairment rather than the genetic difference.

The cervical dystonia has a similar good response to DBS and, together with the primary generalized dystonia, is the most frequent indication for DBS. Cervical dystonia can be focal (i.e., restricted to the neck) or segmental spreading to arms or trunk. Myoclonus dystonia is an inherited disease with myoclonus predominantly in the trunk and dystonia most often cervical or task-specific writer's cramp. In this group, the prevalence of psychiatric problems is high. DBS targeting the GPi improves dystonia in 41–89% and myoclonus in 65–94% of patients. If there is not enough effect on the myoclonus, the implantation of a second electrode in the ventral intermediate nucleus of the thalamus can be considered. Reports show a high incidence of severe psychiatric problems after DBS; however, this could also be a part of the disease. Despite the psychiatric problems, an improvement of quality of life is claimed.

Craniocervical dystonia (Meige's syndrome) and blepharospasm show good results regarding the reduction of blepharospasm, similar to previous findings, but little effect on speech and swallowing. Side effects of bradykinesia have been reported more often in this patient group.

Acquired Dystonia

In general, it is difficult to predict the outcome for acquired dystonia. The effect is more variable than in the group with non-acquired dystonia, but in every subgroup favorable outcomes have been reported. Complicating factors in this group can be the presence of brain lesions, making an operation more challenging; progressive disease; and the presence of other disabling symptoms. Dystonia can occur in different types of neurodegenerative diseases due to progressive brain damage. Only small groups of patients are described. The largest cohort included 24 patients with neurodegeneration with brain iron accumulation, with some positive results but a high variation in response. Dyskinetic dystonic cerebral palsy treated with DBS showed a high variation and a relatively small effect of 15% on BFMDRS. Refractory tardive dyskinesia and dystonia due to medication is a secondary dystonia with a good result on DBS, with a reported improvement of 70–80% on BRMDRS, the Abnormal Involuntary Movement Scale (AIMS), or the Extrapyramidal Symptom Rating Scale (ESRS), and the psychiatric side effects were not different from other indications for DBS.

KEY POINTS TO REMEMBER

- DBS is a treatment option that should be considered in refractory dystonia.
- When considering DBS, it is important to consider the severity of the dystonia, the limitations due to dystonia, and the expected improvement (taking into account the type of dystonia and other disabling symptoms).
- Favorable outcome is seen in primary generalized dystonia, cervical dystonia, and tardive dyskinesia and dystonia.

Further Reading

Fox MD, Alterman RL. Brain stimulation for torsion dystonia. *JAMA Neurol* 2015;72:713–719.

Schjerling L, Hjermind LE, Jespersen B, et al. A randomized double-blind crossover trial comparing subthalamic and pallidal deep brain stimulation for dystonia. *J Neurosurg* 2013;119:1537–1545.

Speelman JD, Contarino MF, Schuurman PR, Tijssen MAJ, de Bie RMA. Deep brain stimulation for dystonia: Patient selection and outcomes. *Eur J Neurol* 2010;17(Suppl 1):102–106.

20 Twists and Turns

Susan H. Fox

You see a 42-year-old woman in your clinic with a
1-year history of posterior neck pain and involuntary
head movement to the left in the past 6 months. Her
background medical history is unremarkable, and she
is on no regular medications. She describes the gradual
onset of a pulling sensation, in addition to movement of
her head during periods of stress or pressure at work.
She had found that touching her chin gently on either
side could help control these movements. Reading
had become bothersome over time as she found it
difficult to control her head with both hands holding
a book. On examination there is a tilt of her head to
the right with rotation of her head to the left, with a
maximum excursion of approximately 30 degrees. She
can intermittently return her chin to a normal position,
but this is followed by a slow drift back to the original
dystonic posture. With her hand gently placed against the
right side of her chin, she can maintain her head in the
neutral position for a longer period of time.

What do you do now?

THERAPEUTIC OPTIONS IN FOCAL DYSTONIA

This patient has an adult onset of a focal neck dystonia without any other neurological condition or cause; thus, this is a primary cervical dystonia. Dystonia is characterized by abnormal postures or movement produced by involuntary muscle contraction, describing in essence the problem encountered by this patient. The identification of dystonic posturing is relatively simple, but it is important to know when to look for underlying causes of a secondary dystonia. Whereas childhood-onset primary dystonia tends to start focally and then spread to become generalized, adult-onset primary dystonia (AOPD) typically starts focally, or in one body part, and remains focal in most cases. In a small proportion of cases, approximately 10–20%, dystonia will spread to an adjacent body part (segmental dystonia). AOPD appears to be an inherited disorder with poor penetrance and an unknown contribution from environmental factors. Mutations in genes more typically associated with primary generalized dystonia, *DYT1* and *THAP1*, can give rise to a focal phenotype, although the low frequency of these mutations in AOPD means routine testing is not warranted. The risk of transmission to children of affected individuals appears to be small, with greater than 75% of patients having an apparently sporadic disease. Onset is typically in the fifth or sixth decade, with some phenotypes tending to start earlier (focal hand dystonia or writer's cramp) and others later (blepharospasm). Secondary dystonia can also present focally, but additional features in the history or examination often help to identify these cases (discussed later).

Diagnosis

The diagnosis of AOPD is purely clinical. Neuroimaging should be normal to make the diagnosis and is not always necessary with a typical history and presentation in the absence of other findings. Neurophysiological testing is generally of no assistance because dystonic muscle contraction looks no different from voluntary muscle contraction on routine electromyography, and all that is seen is the electrical correlate of what is evident clinically. On a research basis, abnormalities of cortical plasticity may be a useful biomarker for primary dystonia, although currently this test is not routinely available. The diagnosis of AOPD can often be made on a first clinic visit if the pattern of movement is consistent, if the age of onset is typical, and if no other neurological abnormalities are found apart from tremor. If an affected body part has a tremor associated with the abnormal posture, as is common in cervical dystonia, the tremor is by convention referred to as a dystonic tremor. If the tremor involves a body part that has no clinical dystonia, such as an upper limb where the dystonia is localized to the neck, the syndrome is referred to as dystonia *with* tremor. This distinction serves little clinical utility, however. The more common phenotypes of AOPD are as follows:

- Cervical dystonia: This is the most common form of AOPD, producing rotational head movement (torticollis), a tilt to one side (laterocollis), forward pulling (anterocollis), or involuntary neck extension (retrocollis). Shoulder displacement or elevation is commonly seen as part of the dystonia or as a compensatory phenomenon. "Spasmodic torticollis" is sometimes used as a general term for cervical dystonia, but not all patients have rotational movement. Most patients have a combination of these postures, with or without tremor. Retrocollis is often associated with prior neuroleptic exposure as a form of tardive dystonia, or even acutely following administration of a dopamine antagonist. Three-fourths of patients will have a sensory trick or *geste antagonistique* whereby superficial cutaneous stimulation can provide temporary relief, a phenomenon not limited to cervical dystonia. Pain is more prominent in cervical dystonia than in other forms of AOPD and in some patients accounts for more disability than the involuntary movement.
- Focal hand dystonia: This can be restricted to writing only, when it is commonly known as writer's cramp. If involving all or a number of different tasks, it is better referred to as focal hand dystonia. It is unclear if these two syndromes are related in terms of pathophysiology. Writer's cramp is one of the so-called "task-specific" dystonias, which have been associated with frequent use or overuse of the involved body part. It is clear, however, that not all people who write for prolonged periods develop dystonia. Patients with writer's cramp can complain of cramping of their hand and commonly experience increasing forearm discomfort as they continue to write. Writer's cramp can develop in the contralateral hand if an effort is made to switch writing hand. A number of other task-specific dystonias other than writer's cramp have been described, and most common are those seen among musicians, such as *embouchure* dystonia seen in those playing wind instruments or task-specific hand dystonia in guitarists.
- Blepharospasm: This commonly presents in older age groups (sixth and seventh decades) and may be associated with a greater risk of spread. Blepharospasm is often preceded by nonspecific sensory symptoms such as "gritty eyes" or "dry eyes," and for this reason patients will often be seen first by an ophthalmologist. The bilateral contraction

of orbicularis oculi muscle can be severe, rendering some patients functionally blind during episodes. The frequency of events can vary considerably, making the diagnosis difficult if no contractions are evident in the clinic. Some patients obtain relief by wearing dark glasses or pressing a finger between their eyes as a form of sensory trick.

- Oromandibular dystonia: This manifests as jaw opening or jaw closure. Some patients have additional deviation to one side. This is a particularly distressing form of focal dystonia because the dystonic contractions can interfere with feeding and communication. Oromandibular dystonia in combination with blepharospasm is known as Meige's syndrome. Like retrocollic cervical dystonia, oromandibular dystonia is often seen in secondary dystonia following neuroleptic exposure, although in tardive dystonia there is often prominent orolingual involvement.
- Laryngeal dystonia: This focal dystonia is also known as spasmodic dysphonia, representing dystonic contraction of the laryngeal muscles responsible for bringing about movement of the vocal cords. In adductor dysphonia, the cords are held tightly together close to the midline, giving the voice a strained strangulated quality. In abductor dysphonia, excessive amounts of air are allowed to pass through the vocal cords, giving a breathy quality to speech.
- Focal lower limb dystonia: This is very rare as a form of AOPD and typically represents a symptomatic dystonia, following basal ganglia infarction, for example. Likewise, hemi-dystonia involving an arm and leg on the same side is typically the result of an underlying lesion, and imaging should be performed in these cases.

Differential Diagnosis

- Parkinson's disease can present with focal foot dystonia in adulthood, particularly in early onset forms that may have a monogenic basis. There may or may not be additional features of parkinsonism in unaffected limbs at the time of first presentation.
- Cervicomedullary lesions can present with a symptomatic cervical dystonia. These are uncommon causes of dystonic posturing but should be considered when there are pyramidal signs in the lower limbs. These lesions can be intramedullary (e.g., gliomas) or extramedullary (e.g., meningioma of the foramen magnum).

- Atlantoaxial subluxation is another uncommon cause of secondary cervical dystonia in adults, tending to present with a fixed limitation of neck movement in children.
- Tics can be difficult to separate from the frequent blinking that can be an early feature of developing blepharospasm. Tics tend to be distractible and dystonia is generally not. Tics are also accompanied by reports of a feeling of tension that is relieved by blinking. Tics are also suppressible, which leads to a buildup of tension or discomfort, features not associated with blepharospasm.
- Functional dystonia: Unfortunately, many patients with organic dystonia were labeled as being hysterical as recently as the 1970. Functional dystonia is diagnosed on the basis of unusual patterns of movement, atypical postures, or unusual distribution of dystonia. Unlike intermittent functional movement disorders such as tremor, functional dystonia does not lend itself to distraction or entrainment, which can make the diagnosis difficult. If suspected, referral to an experienced center is important before embarking on a course of treatment with botulinum toxin (see Treatment section).

Treatment

Oral Drug Therapies

Anticholinergic medications such as trihexyphenidyl, procyclidine, or biperiden are often tried as first-line treatments when symptoms are frequent or troublesome. This class of medication is poorly tolerated in older patients, in whom subjective memory complaints are common. Dry mouth, bladder outflow obstruction, and blurring of vision are all dose-limiting effects of cholinergic antagonism. Where tolerated, even at high doses, the therapeutic effect on abnormal postures is typically small, although tremor can sometimes respond well. Like anticholinergic agents, tetrabenazine is a dopamine-depleting drug used in primary generalized dystonia in children. Its side effect profile also makes it a poor choice for more limited dystonia in adults, with the potential to cause parkinsonism and mood disturbance. Benzodiazepines are often prescribed because they can help with pain and also improve anxiety that can further drive dystonic contractions. Their addictive potential makes them poor long-term options, however, and they are best kept for circumstances in which temporary relief is required.

Botulinum Toxin

The focal nature of AOPD makes it ideal for chemodenervation with botulinum toxin, which is now the gold standard. This treatment is delivered by intramuscular injection and typically lasts 10–12 weeks. Chronic treatment is required because symptoms will return as the biological effect of the toxin recedes. Cervical dystonia also responds well in most patients, but some complex cases need input from an experienced injector to allow optimal muscle selection (Table 20.1). Injections are delivered "blind" or with electromyographic guidance, although there is no strong evidence to support one approach over another except in focal hand dystonia, in which localization is key to prevent the spread of toxin to uninvolved muscle groups and disabling hand weakness. Caution is advised when treating patients with different brands of toxin because there is not unit dose equivalence. Care must be taken when injecting anterior cervical muscles, particularly the sternocleidomastoid muscle bilaterally, because diffusion into pharyngeal muscles can

TABLE 20.1 **Patterns of Cervical Dystonia and Muscles Typically Involved in Producing the Dystonic Movement**

Posture	Muscles to Target with Botulinum Toxin
Torticollis	Contralateral sternocleidomastoid m. Trapezius m. Ipsilateral splenius capitus m.
Laterocollis	Ipsilateral sternocleidomastoid m. Levator scapulae m. Splenius m. Trapezius m. Scalene ms.
Anterocollis	Bilateral sternocleidomastoid m. Digastric m. Anterior scalene m. Platysma m.
Retrocollis	Bilateral splenius m. Semispinalis capitis m. Cervical trapezius m.
Shoulder elevation	Ipsilateral levator scapulae m. Trapezius m.
Tremulous cervical dystonia "No–no" type "Yes–yes" type	Bilateral splenius capitis m. ± sternocleidomastoid m. Bilateral semispinalis capitis m. Sternocleidomastoid m.

give rise to temporary dysphagia; this is typically mild but can be distressing if patients are not warned.

Deep-Brain Stimulation

Deep-brain stimulation is generally reserved for patients with more extensive dystonia involving a number of muscle groups that would be impractical to treat with botulinum toxin. Up to one-third of patients with focal dystonia, however, will have a suboptimal response. In these patients, ongoing disabling pain or dystonic contractions that interfere with function warrant consideration of deep-brain stimulation. Cervical dystonia and Meige's syndrome are the forms of AOPD for which good evidence exists to support the use of bilateral stimulation of the internal globus pallidus. The degree of disability attributable to the focal dystonia must be great enough to warrant the risks of surgery.

KEY POINTS TO REMEMBER

- AOPD occurs in isolation in otherwise healthy adults. The presence of other neurological abnormalities, apart from tremor, precludes the diagnosis and should prompt a search for causes of secondary dystonia.
- Responses to treatment of focal dystonia with oral agents are generally poor, with rare exceptions. Anticholinergics are the main treatment option, and use is limited by side effects. Failure to respond or intolerance warrants early consideration of botulinum toxin.
- A careful history of drug exposures should be taken and clarified with the patient's pharmacy if unclear. Prior neuroleptic exposure is important because focal dystonia can be a manifestation of a tardive syndrome.
- Neck pain is common in cervical dystonia, as is degenerative cervical spine disease. Intractable neck pain not responding to botulinum toxin should be investigated with magnetic resonance imaging of cervical spine, particular if there are radicular features.
- Deep-brain stimulation remains an option for cases refractory to botulinum toxin in which pain or disability is severe enough to warrant acceptance of the surgical risk.

Further Reading

Defazio G, Berardelli A, Hallett M. Do primary adult-onset focal dystonias share aetiological factors? *Brain* 2007;130:1183–1193.

Dressler D. Botulinum toxin for treatment of dystonia. *Eur J Neurol* 2010;17(Suppl 1):88–96.

Stacy M. Epidemiology, clinical presentation, and diagnosis of cervical dystonia. *Neurol Clin* 2008;26(Suppl 1):23–42.

PART V

Other Movement Disorders

21 Delayed and Often Persistent

Susan H. Fox

A 47-year-old woman with schizophrenia is referred
to you with abnormal facial movements and difficulty
walking. She had been taking haloperidol for 10 years.
She was previously on thioridazine for 5 years, but it
was changed to risperidone approximately 8 months
ago due to loss of benefit and sedative side effects.
Six months ago, she started to notice that her mouth
would involuntarily open and she had some neck pulling
backwards. She also feels off balance when walking
and tends to trip easily. She is embarrassed by the facial
movements and wants them to stop. Her psychiatrist does
not want to change the risperidone because she is now
doing much better in terms of psychotic symptoms; the
auditory hallucinations have stopped and she is also now
managing to be more independent and has moved into
her own apartment. On examination, she has involuntary
jaw opening with extension of her neck (retrocollis) and
extension of her back. When she walks, her right foot
turns inwards and her arms invert with extension of the
back. Walking backwards reduces the truncal movements.

What do you do now?

TARDIVE DYSKINESIA

This patient has developed tardive dystonia. Tardive syndromes are drug-induced hyperkinetic movement disorders that occur as a consequence of dopamine D2 receptor antagonism/blockade. There are several types described, and it is important to the management of these disorders that the type of movement disorder induced is identified. The clinical spectrum includes the following:

- *Classical tardive dyskinesia*—repetitive, stereotyped, choreiform oral (chewing), buccal, and lingual movements; rhythmic back-and-forward truncal movements; diaphragmatic contractions with grunting and respiratory noises. Movements are often suppressed by talking and eating.
- *Tardive dystonia*—with more sustained involuntary contraction of orbicularis oculi (blepharospasm); jaw-opening or jaw-closing dystonia; lingual dystonia, neck dystonia (commonly torticollis and retrocollis); truncal hyperextension/tilt ("Pisa syndrome"); intorsion of the arms; limb and foot dystonia. Movements often improve with walking and "sensory trick" (e.g., walking backwards).
- Rarely, *tardive tics, tardive myoclonus, possibly tardive tremor* (but this is more commonly a drug-induced parkinsonism that occurs with bilateral akinesia and rigidity and less commonly a resting limb or jaw tremor)

Tardive syndromes typically occur within 3–6 months of starting a dopamine D2 receptor antagonist, although they may occur within 1 month in elderly patients. Symptoms also frequently occur after stopping a dopamine antagonist, and symptoms can persist for up to 3 months following withdrawal of the offending agent. All antipsychotic drugs are dopamine D2 antagonists, and all have a tendency to induce tardive syndromes. Typical antipsychotics have the highest risk (5% per year) compared to "atypical" antipsychotics (0.5–3% per year). The atypical antipsychotic clozapine has the lowest risk of tardive syndromes (<0.1%). Risk factors for developing tardive syndromes, especially tardive dyskinesia, include older age, female sex, smoking, and diabetes. Tardive dystonia appears to affect younger patients. Patients who are started on an antipsychotic should be monitored for abnormal movements (including drug-induced parkinsonism) prior to starting the drug and every 6 months.

Dopamine D2 antagonists also cause other neurological side effects. These include the following:

- *Parkinsonism*—usually symmetrical slowness (bradykinesia), rigidity, and slow walking; may take up to 3 months to improve on stopping the offending drug.

- *Akathisia*—a subjective report of inner restlessness and inability to sit still, with repetitive stereotyped leg and trunk movements, relieved by moving about; some subjects also have vocalizations.

MANAGEMENT

Ideally, the patient should be switched to an antipsychotic with the lowest propensity to induce tardive syndromes, such as quetiapine or clozapine. However, these atypical antipsychotics can have other bothersome side effects, including metabolic syndrome with weight gain, postural hypotension, and sedation. Clozapine requires mandatory white blood count monitoring due to a minor (<1%) risk of neutropenia. Sometime the symptoms will abate if the antipsychotic that was stopped is restarted. The symptoms will likely return in the future, but this can reduce marked involuntary movements temporarily.

Specific treatments for tardive dystonia include the following:

- Botulinum toxin A for the focal dystonia (i.e., jaw-opening dystonia and neck dystonia; possible in-turning of the right foot). Other types of focal tardive syndromes that can be helped by botulinum toxin A include blepharospasm and jaw-closing dystonia. Tongue injections are not recommended due to the risk of dysphagia.
- Benzodiazepines—clonazepam 0.5–1 mg OD
- Anticholinergics—may reduce tardive dystonia because the mechanism is similar to other dystonia syndromes for which anticholinergics can be helpful. However, side effects limit usefulness; in addition, these agents can exacerbate tardive dyskinesia.
- Tetrabenazine—a central monoamine depletor (dopamine and serotonin) that can reduce hyperkinetic movement disorders. The starting dose is usually 12.5 mg BID or TID, increased to 25 mg TID. The subjects who get the best response usually do so at lower doses. There is a genetic variability in response to tetrabenazine due to its extensive hepatic first-pass metabolism; thus, individual dosing varies between 25 and 75 mg/day. Dose-related side effects include sedation, parkinsonism, and depression. Concomitant use of antipsychotics with tetrabenazine is safe.
- Clozapine—monotherapy with clozapine for treatment-resistant tardive dystonia is often helpful. Side effects include sedation and metabolic syndrome, and blood monitoring is required.
- Other oral medications that have been suggested but for which there is limited evidence or efficacy include clonidine, valproate, levetiracetam, piracetam, beta-blockers, vitamin E, vitamin B$_6$, long branched-chain

amino acids, acetylcholinesterase inhibitors (donepezil, galantamine, and amantadine), and opioid antagonists (naltrexone).

- Surgical options include bilateral globus pallidus internus deep-brain stimulation for treatment-resistant dystonia. This approach has been used in subjects with severe generalized as well as focal dystonia unresponsive to other treatment options.

KEY POINTS TO REMEMBER

- Tardive syndromes can occur with all antipsychotic drugs, including so-called atypical drugs.
- Patients taking these drugs should be evaluated frequently for side effects.
- Evaluating the nature of the movement (i.e., chorea or dystonia) is important because treatment options can differ according to the type of dyskinesia present.

Further Reading

Canadian Psychiatric Association. Clinical practice guidelines: Treatment of schizophrenia. *Can J Psychiatry* 2005;50(13 Suppl 1):7S–57S.

Fernandez HH, Friedman JH. Classification and treatment of tardive syndromes. *Neurologist* 2003;9(1):16–27.

Soares-Weiser K, Fernandez HH. Tardive dyskinesia. *Semin Neurol* 2007;27(2):159–169.

Soares-Weiser K, Rathbone J. Neuroleptic reduction and/or cessation and neuroleptics as specific treatments for tardive dyskinesia. *Cochrane Database Syst Rev* 2006 Jan 25;(1):CD000459.

22 The Stand-Alone Tremor

Robertus M. A. de Bie

A 54-year-old woman visits the clinic because of
bothersome shaking of both hands. The shaking started
slowly when she attended college, aged 16 years, and has
gradually worsened. Now, the tremor hinders her daily
activities. For drinking, she needs to hold a cup with both
hands to avoid spilling. Mostly she uses mugs, which are
half full. She is unable to eat soup with a spoon. She did
not notice shaking of her head, voice, or legs. Sometimes
she drinks one or two glasses of wine before social
meetings because the tremor temporarily subsides. Her
father had a tremor of his head, voice, and hands, and her
elder brother has a tremor of his hands. She knows this is
a family trait, but she wants something to help reduce her
tremor when she is working.

What do you do now?

ESSENTIAL TREMOR

The first step is to review the clinical phenomenology of the tremor to confirm the diagnosis of familial essential tremor.

Tremor

Tremor is an involuntary oscillating movement of a body part. It is the most frequent movement disorder and may be an accompanying symptom in many conditions (Box 22.1).

For the differential diagnosis, it is helpful to ask the following questions regarding the characteristics of the tremor:

- Is there a resting tremor?
- Is there a tremor on holding a posture?
- Is there a tremor when the limb moves?
- Is the frequency of the tremor very low or very high?
- Is it a tremor or are there other involuntary movements such as myoclonus?
- Are accompanying symptoms and signs present, such as dystonia or parkinsonism?

To assess whether the patient has a resting tremor, one needs to be certain that the limb or body part is fully supported and resting or is very loosely hanging. Besides a resting tremor, tremors can occur when the body part is held in a certain position (i.e., postural tremor)—for example, when the patient holds the arms outstretched in front of the chest. The third type of tremor occurs while the limb is moving (i.e., kinetic tremor) or during an intentional action such as

---

BOX 22.1   **Causes of Postural Tremors**

Physiological tremor
Essential tremor
Parkinson's disease
Toxin- or medication-induced tremor
Dystonic tremor
Cerebellar tremor
Task-specific tremor (e.g., writing tremor)
Holmes tremor
Polyneuropathy
Orthostatic tremor
Psychogenic or functional tremor

---

finger pointing or writing (i.e., intention tremor). Another property of tremor is frequency. Because the range of possible frequencies of almost all tremor types is large, and therefore the frequencies of the different tremor types overlap considerably, the frequency in itself is not very helpful for the differential diagnosis. There are two exceptions to this rule. Holmes tremor has a very low frequency of 2–5 Hz; it occurs after stroke and causes rest, postural, and intention tremor. The other tremor with a characteristic frequency is a rare tremor that occurs on standing and goes away on walking called orthostatic tremor of the leg; it has a very high frequency of 13–18 Hz.

Differentiating tremor from other movement disorders is important. Myoclonus is brief, involuntary movements due to muscle jerks or due to brief losses of muscle tone followed by compensatory jerks of the antagonist muscles that can cause a typical "bouncing" stance or flapping hands (i.e., negative myoclonus and asterixis). Occasionally, it may be difficult to distinguish tremor and myoclonus—for example, if the myoclonus occurs very frequently or if the interval between the jerks is almost regular. One example occurs in subjects with multiple system atrophy, in which irregular jerky finger movements may be seen on outstretched hands that are a mixture of tremor and myoclonus. In these cases, a polymyogram with surface electromyography that measures muscle activity can be helpful to distinguish tremor and myoclonus. Symptoms and signs that may be helpful for the diagnostic process are, for example, slowness and stiffness (indicating parkinsonism) and dystonia (e.g., torticollis or hand dystonia).

Essential Tremor Defined

Essential tremor is considered a monosymptomatic disease—that is, the only symptom is tremor. It is defined as long-standing bilateral hand/arm tremor that is visible and may occur persistently during posture holding, simple movements, and intentional actions. The tremor may be slightly asymmetrical. Other areas of the body that may be affected are head and neck (most frequently), the voice, and the legs. Head tremor without limb tremor is accepted as essential tremor, although this definition remains slightly controversial because isolated head tremor could also be considered a manifestation of cervical dystonia, among other disorders. Essential tremor is a progressive disease and manifests at any age, with the mean age being 35 years, but the tremors may also start during childhood. The tremor increases with activities such as drinking from a cup, eating with a spoon, and writing. The size of the handwriting may be normal or larger, in contrast to Parkinson's disease (PD), in which the handwriting is typically smaller. Almost half of the patients have a positive family history for tremors. Although essential tremor is common, to date no gene has been identified as the cause. In 50% of cases, alcohol reduces the tremor. A patient with essential tremor may have a mild gait ataxia during the physical examination, especially late in the disease.

Differential Diagnosis

- PD: Patients with essential tremor do not have postural and gait impairments and have no rigidity, but you may find the cogwheel phenomenon. A "no–no" or "yes–yes" tremor of the head indicates essential tremor, whereas a tremor of the jaw or tongue fits more with PD. Patients with PD may have postural tremors; the tremor starts gradually after some delay. However, this is a re-emerging rest tremor and can also been seen on walking. In contrast, in essential tremor the tremor is present directly when the posture is started and is usually absent when walking.
- Hyperthyroidism
- Toxin- and medication-induced tremors: These are common and often curable—stop the offending medication. Common classes of drugs that cause postural and kinetic tremors include antidepressants, antiepileptics, and chemotherapy agents.
- Exaggerated physiological tremor—anxiety- or caffeine-induced postural tremor
- Dystonic tremor: It is usually very asymmetrical and associated with dystonia in the limb. It is often present at rest as well as postural.

Treatment

In a few patients with essential tremor, the tremor becomes so disabling that they seek medical attention. Treatment with medication is effective in less than 50% of patients and is often unsatisfactory due to bothersome side effects. There does not seem to be a correlation with individuals who respond well to alcohol and treatment options.

The first choice is propranolol. Start with a sustained-release formulation (40–80 mg) once a day (or less). If this is unsatisfactory, increase the dose each week up to a maximum of 320 mg per day. Doses higher than 320 mg per day have not been proven to be more efficacious. Side effects include sedation, postural hypotension, and bradycardia leading to dizziness and occasional syncope. Ask about a history of asthma because this would be a relative contraindication for use of propranolol.

Primidone is a structural analog of phenobarbital. The starting dose of primidone should be low (15 mg per day), taken at bedtime. After 3 days, increase the dose to 15 mg twice a day. Then, increase the dose every third day with 30 mg per day (in two doses) up to, for example, 500 mg per day or until satisfactory tremor reduction is achieved. Primidone is slightly more effective than propranolol, but side effects are also more frequent. Side effects include nausea, vomiting, sedation, vertigo, ataxia, and headache. The risks for these side effects can be reduced if therapy is started at low doses. Rarely, some people have an idiosyncratic reaction to the first dose with severe sedation that precludes further use of the drug. Primidone is a barbiturate with all the issues of tolerance.

If monotherapy with propranolol or primidone is not beneficial but is tolerated, the two agents may be used in combination (rare in the author's experience).

Other agents proposed for essential tremor include gabapentin, topiramate, levetiracetam, benzodiazepines, and mirtazapine. However, based on clinical experience, these agents are usually not very effective. One other option is injecting botulinum toxin into the limb, but the risk of reversible weakness needs to be considered. If medications are not helpful or are tolerated poorly and the tremors are very disabling, treatment with deep-brain stimulation of the thalamus can be considered.

KEY POINTS TO REMEMBER

- Patients with essential tremor have bilateral tremor. Tremor in PD mostly starts unilaterally.
- A no–no or yes–yes tremor of the head indicates essential tremor, whereas a tremor of the jaw or tongue fits with PD.
- You may also find the cogwheel phenomenon in a patient with essential tremor.
- Always rule out toxins and medications as the cause for postural/kinetic tremor.
- Pharmacological options for essential tremor can be unsatisfactory.

Further Reading

Bain P, Brin M, Deuschl G, et al. Criteria for the diagnosis of essential tremor. *Neurology* 2000;54(Suppl 4):S7.

Deuschl G, Raethjen J, Hellriegel H, Elble R. Treatment of patients with essential tremor. *Lancet Neurol* 2011;10:148–161.

23 "She Is So Fidgety"

Robertus M. A. de Bie and Susanne E. M. Ten Holter

A 45-year-old woman presents at the emergency department because she has had progressing uncontrolled movements of the right arm and leg for 1 week. She tells you that she has experienced fatigue for the past few weeks. She has become thirsty and needs to drink a lot of water. She did not have a fever or a throat infection recently. There is no medical history, but she is severely overweighed. She has used oral contraceptive for 15 years and has never used other medications or recreational drugs. Her mother died in a nursing home with dementia, and she did not know her father. On examination, she has hyperkinetic flowing involuntary movement of her arms and legs. The movements worsen when she talks. Her strength is normal, although when asked to squeeze your fingers with her right hand, the grip alternates between tightening and relaxing.

What do you do now?

DEFINING THE MOVEMENT DISORDER

This patient has hyperkinetic involuntary movements that are random and flowing; this would be in keeping with chorea. Choreas are involuntary constant, unpredictable, and unintentional dance-like movements. Patients with chorea are often unaware that they have involuntary movements. Others may try to incorporate the movement into a semipurposeful action (parakinesia). Chorea is usually worse with mental activity or emotion (e.g., talking, mental calculation, or watching a favorite sports team on TV). Physical activity may also exacerbate chorea. The presence of "motor impersistence" is typical of chorea; this is the inability to maintain a posture due to chorea (e.g., protrude the tongue (darting tong) or keep hands in a tight grip (milkmaid's grip)). Sometimes patients can also make unintentional sounds referred to as hyperkinetic dysarthria. Chorea disappears during sleep. Ballism is currently considered a type of chorea with a more proximal distribution and larger movements. It is most often used in the context of hemiballism due to a lesion in the contralateral basal ganglia or cortex. Athetosis is a term formally used for chorea with slow writing movements in the distal limbs. It is not considered a specific entity of chorea anymore.

Differentiating chorea from other hyperkinetic disorders can be difficult. Other hyperkinetic movements are the following:

- Dystonia: Sustained or intermittent involuntary muscle contractions causing abnormal—often repetitive—movements, postures, or both.
- Tics: Random but stereotyped and not usually persistent. They are preceded by an urge and can be temporarily suppressed, whereas chorea cannot be suppressed.
- Myoclonus: Sudden, brief, involuntary muscle jerks due to contraction (positive myoclonus) or interruption of muscle tone (negative myoclonus). These are faster and briefer than chorea, although in children chorea can sometimes be very fast and may resemble myoclonus.
- Pseudo-athetosis: Difficulty keeping a posture due to severely impaired propriocepsis.

FURTHER ANALYSIS

When seeing a patient with chorea, a careful analysis of medical history, family history, and medication use should be made. A full physical examination should be performed to establish whether the chorea is isolated or if other symptoms are present. Pure chorea without any (or very mild) other neurological symptoms is usually a "secondary chorea" such as a chorea due to medications. Chorea

TABLE 23.1 **Common Genetic Causes of Chorea**

Cause	Gene
Autosomal dominant	
Huntington's disease	Huntingtin
Dentatorubropallidoluysian atrophy (DRPLA)	Atrophin 1
Benign hereditary chorea	Thyroid transcription factor 1
Idiopathic brain calcification (Fahr's disease)	
Neuroferritinopathy	Ferritin light chain
Spinocerebellar ataxias (SCA1, -2, -3, -17)	Ataxin 1, 2, 3; TATA-binding protein
Paroxysmal kinesiogenic dyskinesia	Proline-rich transmembrane protein 2 gene (*PRRT2*)
Autosomal recessive	
Chorea acanthocytosis (also XL McLeod's syndrome)	*VPS13A* (chorein)
Pantothene kinase-associated neurodegeneration (PKAN)	Pantothene kinase (*PANK2*)
Also type of neuronal brain iron accumulation (NBIA)	

associated with dystonia, parkinsonism, tics, ataxia, spasticity, abnormal eye movements, and cognitive or personality changes is usually due to a neurode-generative or metabolic process. To establish a genetic cause and to evaluate the pattern of inheritance, the family history can provide important information. However, even in the absence of a positive family history, a genetic cause should not be excluded because it is not always possible to gain a reliable family history (e.g., early death, variable penetrance, symptoms may not be recognized, or the biological parents may not be known). A list of genetic causes of chorea is provided in Table 23.1.

DIFFERENTIAL DIAGNOSIS

In this case the family history was not known, but the course of the symptoms (unilateral and rapid onset), the absence of other neurological deficits, and the accompanying systemic symptoms are clues to an acquired cause. When

BOX 23.1   **Causes of Chorea**

Medications

Dopamine antagonists, antiemetics, lithium
Antiepileptics—phenytoin, valproate
Calcium channel blockers
Levodopa-induced dyskinesia in Parkinson's disease
Stimulants—cocaine, amphetamines
Estrogen (oral contraceptive)
Opiates
Digoxin
Toxins—alcohol, carbon monoxide

Structural Causes

Stroke
Post pump chorea in children
Vascular malformations (e.g., vasculitis, arteriovenous malformation)
Cerebral palsy
Multiple sclerosis
Tumor (lymphoma)

Infections

Meningitis
Viral encephalitis
HIV
Syphilis
Creutzfeldt–Jakob disease

Metabolic

Liver disease—acquired hepatolenticular degeneration (liver failure),
   Wilson's disease
Thyroid
Diabetes—nonketotic hyperglycemia

Autoimmune

Anti-phospholipid antibody in system lupus erythematosis
Chorea gravidarum
Sydenham's chorea (post-streptococcal)
Syphilis
Celiac disease
Paraneoplastic
Anti-Hu, -CRMP5, -Yo, -CV2, -LGI1, -GAD, -CASPR2
Anti-NMDA receptor

Neurodegenerative

Genetic causes (see Table 23.1)
Inherited metabolic disorders

categorized in large groups, causes of "secondary chorea" are infection, autoimmune, paraneoplastic, medication, intoxication, structural causes, metabolic, and neurodegenerative.

Infection, Autoimmune, and Paraneoplastic Causes

The most common cause of chorea in children is Sydenham's chorea, but this can also start in young adulthood and cases in the third decade are described in the literature. Typically, the chorea starts several weeks after a beta-hemolytic streptococcal pharyngitis, and it is thought to be a cross-reaction triggered by anti-streptococcal antibodies that probably target neurons in the basal ganglia. Sydenham's chorea can have a rapid onset, and an asymmetrical presentation is not uncommon. Hypotonia can accompany the disease and may be severely disabling (chorea paralytica), and psychiatric symptoms are often seen (e.g., irritability, outbursts, and obsessive–compulsive symptoms). Other infections that can cause chorea are listed in Box 23.1.

Several autoimmune disorders can be accompanied by chorea. Systemic lupus erythematosus (SLE) and anti-phospholipid syndrome are the most important ones. The etiology is unknown. Other autoimmune disorders in which chorea has been described are Sjögren's syndrome, polycythemia vera, celiac disease, and non-paraneoplastic anti-LGI1 antibodies. The NMDAR encephalitis can be a paraneoplastic syndrome (frequently due to an ovarian teratoma), but it can be an autoimmune syndrome as well. Often there is a broader symptomatology with psychiatric disorders, epilepsy, aphasia, autonomic dysregulation, and eventually coma, but a more benign course is also possible. Other paraneoplastic antibodies that can present with choreatic movements are antibodies against CRMP-5/CV2, Hu, LGI1, Yo, GAD65, and CASPR2.

Chorea gravidarum is chorea during pregnancy. This is more often seen in women with a history of Sydenham's chorea, but other causes, such as SLE, are seen as well.

Medication and Intoxication

A frequent cause of involuntary movements is levodopa in the treatment of Parkinson's disease (generally referred to as levodopa-induced dyskinesia), but chorea can be a side effect of various other medications and this option should always be evaluated. Chorea can also be caused by stimulating recreational drugs (e.g., cocaine and amphetamine) or intoxication (e.g., carbon monoxide and lead). Our patient uses oral contraceptives, but it is less likely that this causes the chorea because she has been using these for 15 years.

Structural Lesions

The most important structural lesion giving acute hemichorea or -ballism is cerebral ischemia. The localization was presumed to be in the subthalamic nucleus; however, case series show a variety of lesions in different basal ganglia nuclei, thalamus, and cortical areas vascularized by the medial cerebral artery.

Metabolic

A metabolic origin of chorea is most often hyperglycemia or hypoglycemia. Computed tomography (CT) shows hyperdense striatal signals, and magnetic resonance imaging (MRI) shows hyperintense striatal signals on T1. Often, patients are diagnosed with diabetes before a period of chorea, but the hyperkinetic movements can be the presenting symptom. The chorea is often reversible by normalization of the blood glucose; sometimes, however, this may take months and symptoms may not resolve completely. Other possible metabolic causes are thyroid disease, vitamin B_{12} deficiency, and parathyroid disorders with disruption of the calcium metabolism. Because these are treatable causes, they should be excluded.

DIAGNOSTICS

It is important to rule out a treatable cause of chorea. This includes a laboratory workup (e.g., blood count, glucose, TSH, vitamin B_{12}, and calcium) and imaging by CT scan or MRI scan. Depending on the disease course, a pregnancy test, antistreptolysin-O, anti-DNAse-B, or paraneoplastic antibodies testing can be considered. If Sydenham's chorea is suspected, a cardial analysis should be performed; if a paraneoplastic disorder is suspected, screening for a primary tumor should be done.

Because Huntington's disease (HD) is the most common cause of genetic adult-onset chorea, genetic testing for it should be considered for all subjects with an adult-onset chorea for which no other secondary cause is found.

BACK TO THE CASE

Laboratory results showed a blood glucose level of 27 mmol/l (486 mg/dl); other results were normal. CT scan showed bilaterally a hyperdense striatal signal that was more prominent on the left side than on the right side. The patient was diagnosed with diabetes mellitus type 2. She was admitted to the hospital and treated for hyperglycemia. Several days after normalization, the chorea disappeared.

TABLE 23.2 Treatment Options for Chorea

Drug (in Order of Suggested Use)	Side Effects
Dopamine antagonists Haloperidol, risperidone, olanzapine, fluphenazine	Tardive syndromes, akathisia, parkinsonism
Tetrabenazine	Parkinsonism, depression, sedation
Amantadine	Livedo reticularis, hallucinations, myoclonus (if renal impairment)
Clozapine	Neutropenia (blood monitoring required), cardiomyopathy (consult cardiologist if tachycardia in rest is present)
Levetiracetam	Sedation, behavioral changes
Riluzole	Weight loss, asthenia, hepatitis, neutropenia (blood monitoring required)

TREATMENT

Depending on the origin of the chorea, the underlying pathology should be treated if possible. For HD, there is no treatment to slow disease progression. Not all individuals need treatment for chorea, and it should be offered only in cases of disabling chorea (Table 23.2). No agent is superior to another, and all carry the risk of potential side effects. In a few reported cases with chorea, deep brain stimulation of the internal part of the globus pallidus has been performed but with a variable effect. It might be necessary to treat accompanying symptoms—for example, in the case of HD, in which mood disorders are frequently present.

KEY POINTS TO REMEMBER

- Chorea has a broad differential diagnosis.
- The most important genetic cause of chorea in adulthood is HD, and genetic testing should be considered as a first step in all patients with adult-onset chorea if no secondary cause is found.
- There are a few treatable and/or reversible causes of chorea that should not be missed.
- Symptomatic treatment is not always necessary.

Further Reading

Chen C, Zheng H, Yang L, Hu Z. Chorea-ballism associated with ketotic hyperglycemia. *Neurol Sci* 2014;35:1851–1855.

Hermann A, Walker RH. Diagnosis and treatment of chorea syndromes. *Curr Neurol Neurosci Rep* 2015;15(2):514.

Mehanna R, Joseph Jankovic J. Movement disorders in cerebrovascular disease. *Lancet Neurol* 2013;12(6):597–608.

Vigliani MC, Honnorat J, Antoine JC. Chorea and related movement disorders of paraneoplastic origin: The PNS EuroNetwork experience. *J Neurol* 2011;258:2058–2068.

Wild EJ, Tabrizi SJ. The differential diagnosis of chorea. *Pract Neurol* 2007;7(6):360–373.

24 "I Have Never Seen Anything Like It Before"

Richard A. Walsh

You meet a 52-year-old woman for assessment of
tremor. Her family doctor is concerned that she may have
Parkinson's disease. On examination she demonstrates
normal facial expression and blink frequency. She speaks
slowly and deliberately. There is an intermittent rest tremor
of her right hand, sometimes characterized by finger
flexion–extension and at other times flexion–extension
movement at the wrist. In addition, there is a high-frequency
tremor of the right leg, with flexion and extension of the
hip. When asked to perform finger movements with the
left hand, the tremor on the right side terminates. Similarly,
slow tongue movements cause the leg and upper limb
movements to break down. When asked to stamp the left
foot to a slower frequency than that seen in the arm and
leg, the right-sided tremor appears to adopt the slower
frequency. There is no true bradykinesia, although all
movements are somewhat effortful and labored. She walks
with her right hand held flexed against her chest.

What do you do now?

FUNCTIONAL MOVEMENT DISORDERS

For the physician without a large amount of experience in the management of tremor disorders, the differentiation and diagnosis of atypical tremor syndromes can be challenging. The textbook 3- to 5-Hz resting tremor of idiopathic Parkinson's disease (PD) that evolves in a classical manner, while keeping the company of the necessary parkinsonian signs to make the diagnosis clear, is rarely problematic. The possibility that tremor can commonly present as a functional movement disorder adds further complexity, and few family physicians will be confident enough to attach a functional label to their patient, preferring the opinion of a specialist clinic. Pattern recognition is of particular importance in tremor, and this is where a specialist's opinion is valuable, although all neurologists should be familiar with the approach to the clinical assessment of functional syndromes which share common phenomenological and historical features. Furthermore, different functional syndromes will often be present in a single patient.

Before discussing the phenomenology of this case, it is important to be clear about terminology. There has been much commentary in the literature in recent years with respect to the most appropriate terms to use when describing movement disorders for which no 'organic' neurological cause can be found. "Psychogenic" and "conversion" disorders are terms commonly used for movement disorders for which an underlying psychological cause is suspected, replacing the older terminology of "hysteria" from the time of Charcot. Some patients will find the term "psychogenic" unacceptable because it appears to suggest an underlying psychological or psychiatric disorder that many of them are unwilling or unable to recognize in themselves, possibly with good reason. This view is supported by the literature and some experts in the field, pointing to no greater prevalence of psychopathology in this patient group compared to the general population. It is also important to recognize that advances in imaging and neurophysiology in this patient group have revealed limited evidence for a physiological disturbance of sensorimotor integration, sometimes in the absence of a demonstrable psychological trigger, making the term "functional" appear more appropriate. It is also less stigmatizing for patients and emphasizes the disturbance in function as opposed to an irreversible or progressive disturbance of structure. Some would argue that the term "functional" flies in the face of the clearly evident dysfunction and sometimes very significant disability experienced by some of these patients.

For consistency, and to follow the trend in the movement disorders literature, the term "functional" is used in this chapter in preference to "psychogenic." In truth, patients presenting with functional movement disorders are less likely to represent a homogeneous cohort with shared pathophysiology and instead represent a common end point for a variety of etiologies, including true disorders of integrative neurobiology, physical manifestations of psychological stress that has no more coherent outlet, and consciously generated movements generated for some form of secondary gain. In some patients, multiple factors may be required, with an appropriate trigger on a susceptible background psychological or genetic substrate.

Diagnosis

Where possible, the diagnosis of a functional movement disorder should be a positive and definitive one based on supportive clinical criteria, with or without laboratory (neurophysiological) support, rather than a diagnosis of exclusion. This shift of emphasis over the past decade has been a subtle but important change that it is hoped will allow for greater efficiency of diagnosis, larger and more uniform patient groups for research, and, perhaps most importantly, confidence on the part of the patient that a correct diagnosis has been made. It would not be uncommon for patients with functional syndromes to go from neurologist to neurologist only to be told emphatically what they "don't have." Such a lack of clarity can perpetuate these conditions and often feeds into the fear of illness that may underpin their genesis in some cases.

There are some general features to the history of a functional movement disorder that will often raise suspicion (Box 24.1), but none of these features are reliable and an emphasis should be placed on the examination. For example, selective disability can be seen in task-specific dystonia and rapid onset can be seen in rapid-onset dystonia parkinsonism, often misdiagnosed as being functional. Tremor is the most commonly encountered form of psychogenic

---

BOX 24.1 **Features on the History That Should Raise Suspicion of a Functional Tremor**

1. Sudden onset, particularly if after emotional or other trivial trauma
2. Selective disability
3. Previous presentations with unexplained neurological symptoms
4. The presence of other possible psychiatric features (e.g., anxiety disorder)
5. Fluctuating course or rapid progression of disability
6. Trauma or injury as a precipitating factor

---

movement disorder, accounting for approximately 50% of cases. A number of changes to these criteria have been proposed, including the addition of a "laboratory-supported, definite" category as suggested by Gupta and Lang, although laboratory support is not a requirement for a positive diagnosis. When available, the neurophysiological assessment of tremor using surface electromyography and accelerometry is a relatively straightforward way of studying tremor frequency and amplitude. Intermittent jerks or movements separated by periods without abnormal movements are amenable to the study of the cortical pre-movement potential or *Bereitshaftspotential*, which, if present, signifies a voluntary basis for the ensuing movement. Unfortunately, few clinicians outside academic centers have access to a neurophysiology laboratory with experience in the study of movement disorders to provide tremor studies as a routine clinical test. Furthermore, the most challenging functional phenotype, functional dystonia, currently has no useful diagnostic neurophysiological test.

The main differential diagnosis for a unilateral tremor includes PD, dystonic tremor, and essential tremor with marked asymmetry. These tremors will of course have their own distinguishing features, with prominence either at rest or with action. Psychogenic tremor typically affects the upper limb more commonly than the lower limb and will often have rest, postural, and action components, sometimes differing in frequency when individually demonstrated but typically of a single frequency when displayed at the same time. Facial, vocal, and tongue involvement is unusual and should prompt exclusion of organic tremor disorders. Likewise, involvement of individual fingers, especially the small abduction–adduction movements seen in polyminimyoclonus, is atypical for psychogenic tremor and should prompt a search for an organic cause. The clinical features that should raise suspicion of a functional tremor are shown in Box 24.2.

BOX 24.2   **Clinical Features in Keeping with a Functional Tremor Disorder**

1. Distractibility
2. Entrainability
3. Inconsistency or variability
4. Coactivation sign
5. Response to suggestion (e.g., application of vibratory stimulus)
6. Keeping company with other atypical features (e.g., convergence spasm and give-way weakness)
7. Increased visual attention to a limb affected by tremor
8. Inconsistent phenomenology
9. Paradoxical worsening with loading

Distractibility

A common error is to presume distractibility is pathognomonic of functional tremors. Distractibility can be seen in dystonic tremor, and the tremor in PD can also be highly variable. Some patients with PD can also exert a certain amount of voluntary control over their tremor. However, distractibility in a patient in whom there are a number of other features suspicious for a psychogenic tremor must be interpreted in the context of the remainder of the examination. Maneuvers commonly employed to demonstrate distractibility include simple conversation or sudden ballistic movements of an uninvolved limb, which can induce a temporary pause in a functional tremor picked up clinically or indeed on surface electromyographic recordings. Complex tasks involving the contralateral limb are particularly effective. Asking the patient to copy a varying pattern of tapping individual fingers against the thumb of the opposite hand, continually pressing for speed and accuracy, is one useful model. Distractibility relies on the often unspoken assumption that there is a significant, if not totally voluntary, generator of functional movements and the associated difficulty inherent in generating and attending to two simultaneous motor tasks.

Entrainment

This examination technique similarly relies on the fact that it is very difficult to voluntarily perform two independent movements at different base frequencies. When a patient with an organic upper limb tremor is asked to perform toe taps of a different frequency, the arm tremor is typically unaffected. This is presumably because the underlying pathophysiological substrate in the cerebellum or basal ganglia is unaffected by the cortical process involved in generating movement elsewhere. In functional tremor, the upper limb tremor will typically fall into coherence or be entrained with the new, imposed rhythm. Essential tremor and parkinsonian tremor involving multiple body parts are typically incoherent. Functional tremor and orthostatic tremor are the only tremor subtypes that demonstrate coherence between body parts. However, some patients with a functional tremor will be able to maintain a different frequency of tremor between hand and foot, a skill employed by some professional musicians. A leg tremor can sometimes voluntarily be locked into an almost clonic rhythm that can resist entrainment. For this reason, the feet should be examined dangling from the side of an examination couch. The closer the entraining rhythm is to the tremor under assessment, the more difficult it is for the tremor (or patient, depending on your view) to resist entrainment. Some patients can be observed to adopt a faster, sometimes very high frequency of tremor in response to an examiner's attempt to entrain, exaggerating the difference in tremor frequency.

Quickly cycling and unpredictable changes in the entraining rhythm, changing from body part to body part, can be useful to aid the diagnosis.

Suggestibility

Functional movement disorders will sometimes be either triggered or relieved by suggestion, and of all the clinical signs, this is one of the most specific. Some practitioners suggest that this form of examination is unethical and aims to "trick" the patient, thereby sacrificing the doctor–patient relationship in the process of making a diagnosis. Many others argue that this type of examination construct is far from administering placebo saline to terminate status epilepticus but, rather, a more subtle, noninvasive, and very safe way to make a positive diagnosis and avoid potentially harmful investigations that may only serve to perpetuate the disorder. In practice, many of us use the principal of suggestibility, if not applying it directly, when taking histories and observing a patient's response to examination.

Patients with an intermittent phenomenon such as jerking movements of a limb can be asked if they can "bring on" an attack, or maneuvers can be performed after a warning that an episode may occur. Alternatively, where a functional movement disorder is constant, such as dystonic posturing or tremor, the examiner can apply a stimulus in an attempt to modulate the underlying cause. This can be pressure applied to the skull or spine of a vibratory stimulus such as a tuning fork. A positive response to this kind of approach can be a positive predictive factor for a good outcome following psychotherapy. More entrenched cases will often fail to respond.

Coactivation Sign

This sign was described and best appreciated during recording from surface electrodes but can also be appreciated in its clinical correlate. Electromyography in a functional wrist tremor identifies a period of tonic coactivation of wrist extensors and flexors at the initiation of tremor, typically lasting less than 300 ms, before an alternating pattern of contraction follows. Clinically, this is picked up as a resistance to passive movement of the involved joint that breaks down with disappearance of the tremor with distraction, unlike true rigidity in parkinsonism, which is sustained or even increased with distracting maneuvers.

PATHOPHYSIOLOGY

The conventional wisdom that functional movement disorders arise from some underlying and unexpressed psychological or emotional trauma is not borne out by the available epidemiological data. These patients do not demonstrate rates of psychiatric comorbidity that are higher than expected in the general population. Of course, an unexpected paucity of reported anxiety or depression does not mean an absence of these conditions. Some authors have demonstrated a high rate of alexithymia, or an impairment of emotional processing at a cortical level, in patients with functional illness. This may explain the failure to demonstrate a higher prevalence of psychopathology in these patients and also offers an interesting avenue for research into the factors that may lead emotional stress to find an alternative avenue of expression though aberrant movements.

There is also evidence that these patients, or at least a subset of them, have dysfunction of sensorimotor integration that interferes with the normal appreciation of performed movement as being volitional, instead interpreting it as involuntary. Self-completed diaries from patients with functional tremor show that they tend to overestimate the duration of their tremor compared to tremor recordings by approximately 65%, compared to approximately 30% in patients with organic tremor. This again suggests a disturbance of sensory perception or feedback in these patients. Functional neuroimaging has demonstrated increased connectivity between limbic areas and the supplementary motor area, possibly implying a maladaptive influence of emotional processing on the planning and performance of voluntary movement. Some patients, on the other hand, have clear social stressors that can be linked to the onset of their symptoms. It is likely a very heterogeneous population that presents with functional movement disorders, with no clear unifying feature other than abnormal movements as the final common pathway.

MANAGEMENT

Although there has been a very positive move toward tackling the diagnostic process and some interesting early progress in unraveling the underlying pathophysiology in functional movement disorders, a consistent and successful approach to management has been elusive. One of the greatest challenges relates to the fact that these patients often fall between the two stools of neurology and psychiatry. Changes in the fifth edition of the *Diagnostic and Statistical Manual of Mental Disorders* (*DSM-5*) may go some way to alleviating the challenge involved when trying to classify these patients, particularly those who deny any symptoms to support an active psychiatric condition. This change removes the requirement to demonstrate psychological factors at the time of diagnosis and places an appropriate emphasis on the neurological examination.

Many patients with functional movement disorders will have been to a number of different neurologists. It is without doubt that the more prolonged the symptomatology, the greater the challenge to reverse maladaptive and deeply ingrained behaviors. Poor communication of the diagnosis can lead to breakdown in the doctor–patient relationship at huge detriment to the patient and the prospect of recovery. It is important to consider psychological factors, even in patients who protest the loudest against the suggestion of stress, and this needs to be addressed as part of a multidisciplinary approach. There are a few principles, although without evidence, that if followed may improve the chance of a good outcome:

- Emphasize that there is no structural abnormality of the nervous system. Ask if any particular illness was a concern so that it can be positively excluded without doubt.
- Ensure that patients understand that no one has said they are "mad" or that their symptoms are "in their head." Acknowledgment that symptoms are no less real than those seen in stroke or epilepsy can offer some validation and help build a therapeutic relationship.
- Reiterate that although the symptoms are very real, they do have the potential to resolve completely given the proven integrity of the nervous system. Patients sometimes appreciate the analogy of an intact computer that has temporarily malfunctioning software.
- Many patients will deny any underlying psychological disturbance. It is useful to highlight the complexity of our personalities and characters and the importance of life experiences in making us who we are. An understanding of this complexity often helps patients accept the need for input from a psychiatrist.
- A close working relationship with a psychiatrist who has experience in the management of patients with neurological disease is crucial. The term "neuropsychiatrist" is also acceptable to patients and again places emphasis on the interaction between motor and emotional centers.

As with all functional disorders, it is important to minimize unnecessary investigations to prevent reinforcing the behavior and the maladaptive response to perceived disability. Likewise, pharmaceutical treatments intended for organic disease must be avoided so that confusing signals are not sent to the patient. A strong emphasis on physical therapies can be successful, although no randomized trials of treatments in psychogenic movement disorders are available. Drug treatment of any coexistent depression or anxiety disorder is clearly warranted when it is believed to be contributing. Involvement of a psychologist or psychiatrist interested in functional movement disorders is valuable in helping to train patients to interpret their emotions and to foster the development of coping strategies where appropriate. Because of the wide heterogeneity of presentations and complexity of patient backgrounds, an individualized approach should be followed.

KEY POINTS TO REMEMBER

- Functional movement disorders are not diagnoses of exclusion. Well-described clinical features on examination, differing among the various functional phenotypes, can allow a positive diagnosis to be made early while avoiding unnecessary investigations.
- It is now recognized that psychiatric or psychological factors need not be present at the time of presentation to make a diagnosis of functional disease, as established in the *DSM-5*. This facilitates the diagnosis and may allow closer and valuable involvement from psychiatry colleagues. However, it is critical that the neurologist remain central to provide an examination focused diagnosis.
- These patients can be hugely complex and their backgrounds often include multiple investigations and different diagnoses. A coordinated multidisciplinary approach is essential.
- The longer the symptom duration, the lower the success rate in resolving functional syndromes. If a diagnosis can be made early in the course of a functional syndrome, it is worthwhile applying as many of the available resources as possible early and often to improve remission rate. Occasionally, focused inpatient therapy is the best way to achieve this goal.

Further Reading

Czarnecki K, Hallett M. Functional (psychogenic) movement disorders. *Curr Opin Neurol* 2012;25:1–5.

Deuschl G, Köster B, Lücking CH, Scheidt C. Diagnostic and pathophysiological aspects of psychogenic tremors. *Mov Disord* 1998;13(2):294–302.

Edwards MJ, Bhatia K. Functional (psychogenic) movement disorders: Merging mind and brain. *Lancet Neurol* 2012;11:250–260.

Espay AJ, Lang AE. Phenotype-specific diagnosis of functional (psychogenic) movement disorders. *Curr Neurol Neurosci Rep* 2015 Jun;15(6):32.

Gupta A, Lang AE. Psychogenic movement disorders. *Curr Opin Neurol* 2009;22:430–436.

Stone J. Functional neurological disorders: The neurological assessment as treatment. *Pract Neurol*. 2016 Feb;16(1):7–17.

25 Slow with an Altered Sensorium

Richard A. Walsh

A colleague has asked for a second opinion on a patient under his care. He is concerned about an atypical parkinsonism. The patient is 72 years of age and has come from home to the emergency department amid reported family concerns about his reduced mobility and cognitive slowing. There is no personal or family history of a movement disorder or dementia. He has experienced intermittent anxiety symptoms throughout his adult life. He has a granddaughter with Tourette's syndrome and behavioral difficulties who moved in with him and his wife 3 months ago, causing considerable stress.

Your colleague noted striking general body bradykinesia and bradyphrenia with a slow stooped gait and what was believed to represent rigidity. On your assessment there is little or no spontaneous speech output and no eye contact. Some questions you ask are repeated. There is no tremor. There is paratonia in the upper limbs. Gait is slow with reduced arm swing, and pull test is positive.

What do you do now?

CATATONIA

Catatonia is a nonspecific syndrome of psychomotor disturbance characterized by motor dysfunction and behavioral change. Catatonia is most often seen in the context of psychiatric illness, but it is also a potential complication of medical disorders associated with a central nervous system (CNS) insult, including infective, traumatic, toxic, and metabolic etiologies. In the past, this syndrome was often associated with schizophrenia; however, due to the advent of successful neuroleptic therapy during the past half century, this association is less common but persists. As with many syndromes, there is a spectrum of severity and milder forms of catatonia as represented here, also known as simple or benign catatonia, are undoubtedly underrecognized, particularly in patients on general medical wards where physicians are less familiar with it. Unfortunately, patients with catatonia may fall between two stools, with psychiatrists sometimes deferring to medical colleagues in the setting of pyrexia and autonomic instability and medical physicians relying on their psychiatry colleagues when there is a prominent psychiatric background and prodrome. Close collaboration is key.

Malignant catatonia represents the most severe end of the clinical spectrum and is marked by its high mortality rate prior to the routine use of electroconvulsive therapy (ECT) in this setting. Fortunately, the high mortality rates of greater than 70% prior to the advent of modern drug therapy of psychiatric disease no longer occur, although the condition remains potentially lethal.

Malignant catatonia can have hyperactive and stuporous phases. There may be a prodrome of agitation and irritability for a number of weeks followed classically by a period of intense motor activity with some or all of the following: hyperthermia, tachycardia, hypertension with anorexia, and reduced oral intake. This period then gives way to stupor and rigidity and life-threatening autonomic instability. Malignant catatonia is a common feature with two drug-induced conditions: neuroleptic malignant syndrome and serotonin syndrome. In their fullest clinical forms, all are associated with alteration of consciousness, autonomic instability, and increased muscle tone. Hyperpyrexia can also be a feature in severe cases of all three conditions. Importantly, the group of patients most associated with a risk of catatonia of any type—that is, patients with psychiatric disease—is also the group most likely to be on treatments placing them at risk of these conditions. Therefore, it is crucial for physicians dealing with these patients to have a good working knowledge of these syndromes and

- Catalepsy—maintenance of uncomfortable positions and postures against gravity
- Waxy flexibility—even and constant resistance to passive induction of postures
- Stupor—absence or paucity of response to external stimuli
- Agitation, not influenced by external stimuli
- Mutism—little or no verbal response with an absence of an alternative explanation
- Negativism—oppositional responses to external instructions or stimuli
- Mannerisms—unusual performances of normal actions or gestures
- Stereotypies—repetitive, frequent, non-goal-directed motor activity
- Echolalia—perseverative repetition of words uttered by someone else
- Echopraxia—perseverative repetition of actions observed in another person

features that may help distinguish between them. Some of the classical clinical signs that can be observed in catatonia are provided in Box 25.1.

INVESTIGATIONS AND DIFFERENTIAL DIAGNOSIS OF CATATONIA

Any medical condition that can produce an altered sensorium and disturbance of motor function can approximate the clinical features of catatonia. Careful observation, a good collateral and drug history, and an early broad screen for mimicking infective and metabolic disorders should minimize the risk of making an error. The following sections present diagnostic considerations that are important to keep in mind, and clues to discriminating each from catatonia of any type are provided.

Neuroleptic Malignant Syndrome

Some authors have suggested that this could be considered an iatrogenic form of catatonia given the similarities in presentation and an attractive hypothesis of dopaminergic hypoactivity that unifies them. Clearly, the distinction is only challenging where catatonic features develop while on a neuroleptic. For this reason, discontinuation of the neuroleptic is advised in this setting to remove any confusion and as a potentially therapeutic step for neuroleptic malignant syndrome (NMS). Development of hyperpyrexia prior to onset of stupor may be a useful indication of NMS over catatonia when hyperpyrexia can be observed in the hyperexcitable phase where one exists.

Serotonin Syndrome

Serotonin syndrome is a toxic serotoninergic state caused by substances that reduce the breakdown or increase the release of serotonin within the CNS. Again, a good drug history is key, and do not hesitate to contact pharmacies or relatives to confirm what may be inaccuracies recorded in the emergency department. Serotonin syndrome is characterized by neuromuscular hyperexcitability more than rigidity, and clonus and spasticity in the lower limbs are suggestive signs. Auscultation of abdominal bowel sounds, often neglected, can support serotonin syndrome where found to be hyperactive.

Acute Dopaminergic Withdrawal State

Patients with Parkinson's disease are particularly vulnerable at the time of emergency admission to the hospital with acute medical illness. When presenting with aspiration pneumonia, stroke with compromised swallow, or when in intensive care scenarios, the omission of oral dopaminergic therapy is unfortunately not uncommon and the consequences can be devastating. The clinical features of what is sometimes known as Parkinson's disease hyperpyrexia syndrome or neuroleptic malignant-like syndrome are similar to NMS, although recovery can be more prolonged given the associated comorbidities. Rapid institution of levodopa via nasogastric intubation may be required, or if the enteric route is not available, apomorphine or transdermal rotigotine can be used. A past history of Parkinson's disease, if available, should make the distinction from catatonia relatively easy, although patients with Parkinson's disease may be a high risk group for catatonia given the background dopaminergic deficit.

Akinetic Mutism

Like catatonia, the akinetic mute state is a final common end point for a number of diverse pathologies. The two syndromes also share anatomic localization with akinetic mutism being seen in disorders that involve the mesencephalo–thalamic region bilaterally (e.g., venous infarction and prion disease) or bilateral frontal lobes (supplementary motor area in particular) such as post-traumatically or following bilateral anterior circulation strokes. In akinetic mutism, rigidity is not a feature and autonomic instability is not typically a feature. There is also retention of consciousness and reactivity to external stimuli, although the nature of responses is slow and spontaneous verbal output is greatly diminished.

NMDA Receptor Encephalitis

This immune-mediated encephalopathy undoubtedly accounted for some cases treated as catatonia prior to its identification in 2007 by Dalmau and colleagues, and it could be considered a medical cause of catatonia given the similarities. This syndrome presents with a psychiatric prodrome of behavioral disturbance with agitation and irritability, with subsequent neuropsychiatric features including paranoia and psychosis. Neurological features including seizures and a state of stupor with autonomic instability ensue. The clinical picture, described as "wakeful unresponsiveness," is of a patient lying with eyes open and sometimes mumbling incoherently. In the final phase, the movement disorder features are prominent and so characteristic to be of use in making the distinction with respect to catatonia. Any of the following can be seen: bruxism, orofacial dyskinesia, stereotyped movements such as hip thrusting, limb dystonia, and chorea. The diagnosis can be confirmed with identification of the antibody in cerebrospinal fluid (CSF) and response to immunosuppression.

Minimally Convulsive Status Epilepticus

It is never an error to consider complex partial or minimally convulsive status epilepticus as a cause of reduced motor and verbal output. This syndrome is readily excluded with an urgent bedside electroencephalography (EEG), which should be able to exclude epileptiform discharges as a cause of obtundation. Notably, seizure activity and catatonia can respond to intravenous lorazepam, although after prolonged subclinical seizure activity a post-ictal state will be expected.

INITIAL INVESTIGATIONS

Although both primary psychiatric etiologies are common, the exclusion of medical causes that might require specific therapy should be the priority. The basic principles of resuscitation should of course apply for any acutely unwell patient. Intravenous fluids, cardiovascular assessment, and monitoring of urine output in severe cases may be necessary. All patients should have liver, renal, and thyroid profiles checked with a full blood count and septic screen. Serum creatinine kinase should be determined to search for evidence of rhabdomyolysis and, if elevated, urine should be tested for myoglobin. An EEG should be performed where seizure activity is a diagnostic possibility. Neuroimaging and CSF analysis should also be considered on a case-by-case basis.

TREATMENT OF CATATONIA

Once the patient is clinically stable and a diagnosis of catatonia is clinically established, close and regular involvement of a psychiatrist familiar with the condition
is essential, particularly when a patient is not being cared for on a psychiatry
ward. Response or "reactivation" following administration of benzodiazepines
is a common clinical feature in cases on the benign end of the spectrum such
as this patient, and this can be a useful diagnostic step when uncertainty exists.
Intravenous lorazepam can be administered initially (1–4 mg iv) when a patient's
medical comorbidities do not preclude it. Observation for respiratory compro-
mise is crucial, and the availability of oxygen and resuscitation equipment should
be confirmed. If effective, the patient should demonstrate more normal motor
activity within 30–60 seconds and may immediately demonstrate a resolution
of stupor with appropriate verbal output. Regular oral lorazepam in high doses
titrated to tolerability (e.g., 1 or 2 mg QDS to start) can then be initiated, and
most patients will demonstrate recovery over a 2-week period. Failure to achieve
any response after 4 or 5 days of benzodiazepine treatment should prompt consideration of electroconvulsive therapy (ECT). In malignant catatonia, ECT may
be required regardless, and this decision should be taken following discussion
with the multidisciplinary team and the patient's family. Even where a transient
response to lorazepam is observed in malignant catatonia, early institution of
ECT may be necessary to precipitate a sustained remission to allow normal oral
intake and avoidance of the potentially fatal medical complications.

Thromboprophylaxis should be instituted as per local guidelines given the
risk of deep venous thrombosis and pulmonary embolism. Assessment by a di-
etitian and speech and language therapist is important to establish adequate and
safe caloric intake. Mobilization with physiotherapy will work toward minimiz-
ing the complications of immobility.

Neuroleptic therapy should be discontinued in patients presenting in a catatonic state. This is because neuroleptics may worsen the negative features of
catatonia and the main differential diagnosis is a neuroleptic malignant syndrome. There are some reports of success with the use of clozapine; however,
expert psychiatrist input is recommended before the reintroduction or initiation
of antipsychotic therapy.

OUTCOME IN THIS CASE

This patient had a benign catatonia, believed to be triggered by the stress and anxiety associated with the complex social issues at home. His family was able to give
a very clear history of normal function in the months prior to his presentation.

He had become agitated and irritable with some psychotic features and reduced self-care in the weeks prior to presentation. He was treated with an intravenous dose of 2 mg lorazepam, which produces excessive sedation. A regular oral dose of 1.5 mg four times daily is tolerated and results in a striking improvement to baseline within 5 days. Maintenance anxiolytic therapy with mirtazapine and low-dose quetiapine were started by the psychiatry service prior to discharge.

KEY POINTS TO REMEMBER

- Catatonia is a syndrome of altered consciousness and psychomotor retardation as a consequence of one of a diverse range of psychiatric and neuromedical disorders. The common pathophysiology may be associated with reduced dopaminergic activity within the frontal–subcortical circuitry.
- Catatonia is uncommon and if not thought of will be easily missed, particularly in its milder forms as in this case. The condition is generally partially or completely responsive to benzodiazepines, which are worth considering as a therapeutic trial when it is a diagnostic possibility.
- Malignant catatonia represents the most severe form of the condition and is a medical emergency that is still fatal in some cases, despite modern psychiatric treatments and intensive care support.
- The main differential diagnosis to consider is neuroleptic malignant syndrome in patients who develop symptoms while receiving neuroleptics for a primary psychiatric illness. All neuroleptics should be discontinued when catatonia is suspected.
- Cooperation and close liaison between psychiatry, neurology, general medical, and anesthetic teams are crucial to ensure every facet of this condition receives subspecialty care to reduce morbidity and mortality from this condition.

Further Reading

Ellul P, Choucha W. Neurobiological approach of catatonia and treatment perspectives. *Front Psychiatry* 2015 Dec 24;6:182.

Wijemanne S, Jankovic J. Movement disorders in catatonia. *J Neurol Neurosurg Psychiatry* 2015 Aug;86(8):825–832.

Wilcox JA, Reid Duffy P. The syndrome of catatonia. *Behav Sci (Basel)* 2015 Dec 9;5(4):576–588.

26 "It Has to Be Functional!"

Richard A. Walsh

You have assessed a 29-year-old woman in your movement disorders clinic for the first time, following a referral for long-standing "cramping" of her feet. This symptom was first experienced at 17 years of age and is described as an "in-turning" of the right foot, fixed or with additional continuous writhing movement, in the absence of pain. Episodes are more likely in the context of fatigue or stress. The movement is described as involuntary and tends to develop after exertion of approximately 30 minutes and resolves with rest after 20 minutes to 1 hour. Between episodes, lower and upper limb function is reportedly normal. Screening questions reveal episodic migraine only.

On enquiry about family history, you are told that her mother had a similar complaint in early adulthood. She is now 65 years of age and no longer has any movement difficulty.

Neurological examination is normal and you are unable to induce any abnormality by asking her to walk up and down the corridor repeatedly.

What do you do now?

PAROXYSMAL EXERCISE-INDUCED DYSKINESIA

Although there are a number of episodic or intermittent movement disorders, when hearing the term "paroxysmal," most neurologists will assume the conversation is about one of three rare primary paroxysmal dyskinesias (PxDs). These movement disorders are very uncommon, rarely seen even by those working in specialist movement disorders clinics. Despite this, many neurologists will have a superficial knowledge about the PxDs due to their interesting phenomenology and recent advances in their genetic and phenotypic characterization.

The clinical picture, based on the original classification system proposed by Demirkiran and Jankovic in 1995, is described in the following section. All categories may demonstrate one or more of the following: dystonia, chorea, and ballism. Triggers, duration of attacks, and response to treatment are more discriminating than age of onset or phenomenology. The three phenotypes, in order of reducing prevalence, are paroxysmal kinesigenic dyskinesia (PKD), paroxysmal nonkinesigenic dyskinesia (PNKD), and paroxysmal exercise-induced dyskinesia (PED). An originally described fourth phenotype known as paroxysmal nocturnal dyskinesia has been removed from this classification, having been definitively recategorized as a form of nocturnal frontal lobe epilepsy. Although a useful construct for researchers and clinicians (Table 26.1), this classification system belies a greater complexity that has begun to emerge with the greater genetic and clinical description of cases worldwide. Some patients with a gene linked to one form of PxD may also manifest the other two phenotypes, some genes associated with one phenotype (e.g., *PRRT2*) can give rise to another in isolation, and the majority of cases identified have no genetic etiology or causative pathology identified at all.

CLASSIFICATION OF PAROXYSMAL DYSKINESIAS

Paroxysmal Kinesigenic Dyskinesia

PKD has been linked with mutations in the *PRRT2* gene and is the most common of the genetic primary paroxysmal dyskinesias. Patients present in childhood with frequent and short-lived episodes of dyskinesia (<1 minute typically) triggered by particular movements, such as rising from a sitting position or gait initiation. Patients will typically get a good result from carbamazepine, with full resolution by the time adulthood is reached in many cases.

Paroxysmal Nonkinesigenic Dyskinesia

Age of onset is variable and has been described throughout life. PKND has been linked to what was known as the myofibrillogenesis regulator 1 gene and now

TABLE 26.1 **Key Clinical Features of the Paroxysmal Dyskinesias by Phenotype**

Phenotype	Age of Onset (Years)	Triggers	Duration of Attacks (Minutes)	Frequency	Distribution	Treatment
PKD	<18	Movement, intention to move	<1	Daily	Generalized	Carbamazepine and other AEDs
PNKD	<18	Caffeine, alcohol, stress, emotion	5–30	Weekly to monthly	Focal, hemibody or generalized	Trigger avoidance, benzodiazepines
PED	<18	Prolonged exercise, fatigue	5–60	Daily to weekly	Focal, lower limbs	Poor response Clonazepam Ketogenic diet?

AEDs, antiepileptic drugs; PED, paroxysmal exercise-induced dyskinesia; PKD, paroxysmal kinesigenic dyskinesia; PNKD, paroxysmal nonkinesigenic dyskinesia.

known as the *PKND* gene. Episodes are less frequent but longer lasting, up to 1 hour in some cases and occasionally longer. Movement is not a trigger, with most attacks being spontaneous, but there are associations with caffeine, stress, and alcohol consumption in some patients.

Paroxysmal Exercise-Induced Dyskinesia

In 30% of cases, PED is associated with mutations in the solute carrier family 2, member 1 (*SLC2A1*) gene on chromosome 1p34.2, which plays a role in glucose transport into the central nervous system via the glucose transporter-1 (GLUT-1). A more severe infantile-onset phenotype of GLUT-1 deficiency is associated with microcephally, seizures, severe developmental delay, and hyperkinetic movement disorders. The phenotype has expanded to include other episodic conditions, epilepsy and migraine, which may coexist with the paroxysmal dyskinesia. The majority of cases have no such association and are either sporadic or familial linked to genetic factors as yet unidentified.

As in this case, hyperkinetic movement in childhood or early adult-onset GLUT-1 deficiency causing PED is typically dystonia in the exercised limb, and it is associated with long periods of exercise.

DIFFERENTIAL DIAGNOSIS

Early Onset Parkinson's Disease Due to a *Parkin* Mutation (*PARK2*)

Primary foot dystonia is uncommon but often seen as a presenting symptom in early onset Parkinson's disease, particularly when associated with *PARK2* mutations. Onset is typically in the context of exertion. This is sometimes mistaken for paroxysmal dystonia associated with GLUT-1 deficiency but should be possible to differentiate on the basis of a number of features. Age of onset in PED is rarely after age 18 years, and in monogenetic Parkinson's disease, onset is rarely before age 18 years. In Parkinson's disease, one would hope to identify some early features of bradykinesia and rigidity inter-ictally, although these could be too subtle in early onset cases. In PED, further periods of exercise of similar duration may not trigger foot dyskinesia, although in Parkinson's disease the onset will be reasonably reliable (before treatment), with recurring onset on repeated exertion. Patients with treated early onset PD that presents with unilateral foot dystonia can go on to develop levodopa-induced dyskinesia on the same side. Before treatment, however, the phenotype is dystonic, whereas in PED there is commonly a choreic or choreodystonic phenotype.

Dopa-Responsive Dystonia

Dopa-responsive dystonia (DRD) is another uncommon condition, which will be on the radar of most neurologists when presented with a young patient with foot dystonia. The diurnal variability and long protracted periods of dystonia lasting hours in the latter half of the day do not support a diagnosis of PED. Some patients with DRD due to GTP-cyclohydrolase mutations will have pyramidal signs in the lower limb, not seen in PED. A trial of levodopa is a useful diagnostic test with a striking benefit in DRD, not expected in PED although reported in a small number of cases in the literature.

Functional Paroxysmal Dyskinesia

It is a certainty that patients with one of the paroxysmal dyskinesias described previously were diagnosed with functional movement disorders in the past and, it is hoped, to a lesser degree today. The paroxysmal and bizarre nature of the movements seen in PED unfortunately make this error inevitable. For functional PxD, the same red flags exist as for other functional disorders. For example, shared company with other somatic complaints without medical explanation, association with litigation or injury, and selective disability and inconsistent or atypical phenomenology should raise clinical suspicion.

Tonic Spasms in Multiple Sclerosis

In demyelination of the central nervous system there can be sudden, paroxysmal stiffening of a limb, which is termed a tonic spasm. Clearly, in the context of a diagnosis of multiple sclerosis, tonic spasms are easily recognized. However, the author has seen this as a presenting feature of multiple sclerosis with isolated spams occurring for years before a diagnosis is made. This is believed to be due to cphaptic transmission between neural tracts injured by demyelination. Episodes are typically very brief, lasting only seconds and therefore typically even shorter than the episodes seen in PKD. There are no triggers, but bouts are possibly more common during illness. Unlike in PED, in which there is lower limb predominance, tonic spasms are more commonly seen in the upper limb in multiple sclerosis and this presumably relates to the prevalence of cervical spine demyelination. Notably, both PKD and tonic spams can respond well to carbamazepine.

TREATMENT OPTIONS

In the small number of cases reported in the literature, the good response to clonazepam makes this a reasonable first therapeutic option. Unlike PKD and

PNKD, PED does not demonstrate the same gratifying response to carbamazepine. A trial of other benzodiazepines and acetazolamide would appear reasonable and low risk, with a low threshold for discontinuation if unhelpful. There are a small number of reports of benefit from levodopa and a ketogenic diet, but the underlying mechanism of the apparent response to these approaches is unknown.

KEY POINTS TO REMEMBER

- The primary paroxysmal dyskinesias are a clinically and genetically heterogeneous group of movement disorders characterized by episodes of hyperkinetic involuntary movements of variable duration and frequency.
- Three genes have been discovered to date that are associated with one or more of three broad phenotypic groups: paroxysmal kinesigenic dyskinesia, paroxysmal nonkinesigenic dyskinesia, and paroxysmal exercise-induced dyskinesia.
- Many patients with a typical phenotype will not be found to have a mutation in one of the three genes identified to date, suggesting the existence of additional genetic associations that remain undiscovered.
- All of the genes described have been shown to have additional neurological associations that include hemiplegic migraine and episodic ataxia.
- Paroxysmal kinesigenic dyskinesia responds well to carbamazepine therapy.

Further Reading

Bhatia KP. Paroxysmal dyskinesias. *Mov Disord* 2011;26(6):1157–1165.

Erro R, Sheerin UM, Bhatia KP. Paroxysmal dyskinesias revisited: A review of 500 genetically proven cases and a new classification. *Mov Disord* 2014 Aug;29(9):1108–1116.

Gardiner AR, Bhatia KP, Stamelou M, et al. PRRT2 gene mutations: From paroxysmal dyskinesia to episodic ataxia and hemiplegic migraine. *Neurology* 2012;79(21):2115–2121.

Gardiner AR, Jaffer F, Dale RC, et al. The clinical and genetic heterogeneity of paroxysmal dyskinesias. *Brain* 2015;138(Pt 12):3567–3580.

27 Could It Possibly Be … ?

Susan H. Fox

A 43-year-old woman presents with a 1-year history of right foot tremor. She has noticed this when sitting with her leg hanging over a couch or bed. She also has some tremor when resting her foot on the pedal while driving. She sometimes feels mild pulling on her big toes at the same time as the tremor. Her general practitioner is concerned because she also seems to have a reduced facial expression. Because she was adopted, there is no known family history of a movement disorder. She is otherwise well and has no functional disability. On examination, her neurological and general exam is normal apart from a low-frequency, irregular foot tremor when sitting and lying and some extensor posturing in her big toe and tremor in her big toe bilaterally. Her walking appeared normal.

What do you do now?

METABOLIC DISORDERS OF CHILDHOOD PRESENTING
WITH MOVEMENT DISORDERS IN ADULTHOOD

The first step is to classify the movement disorder. Further careful examination may be required. This patient has a unilateral resting and possibly postural foot tremor with big toe dystonia, with little else on examination. The position of the leg when examining is important. Pure rest tremor is seen on lying down with leg completely relaxed. Postural leg tremor can be seen in the whole leg when the person is sitting in a chair. In addition, elevation of the leg while lying may bring out postural tremor. Dangling the legs over a high couch so the feet do not touch the ground is probably more in keeping with rest position, but she may not be completely relaxed. On careful observation, she is noted to have tremor in the dystonic toe. Sometimes tremor can be delayed; thus, observing for several minutes in each position is important so as not to miss tremor.

The differential diagnosis of tremor and dystonia is reviewed in Box 27.1 (see also Chapter 17, Table 17.1). In this age group, the most common diagnosis to consider is idiopathic Parkinson's disease (PD). Patients can present with isolated foot or leg tremor, although these are much less common than arm tremor. The average age of onset in tremor-dominant PD is slightly younger than that for non-tremor-dominant PD, possibly reflecting the likely genetic component to the disease. Genetic parkinsonism especially due to *parkin* gene mutations is more likely to have leg tremor. The association with dystonia is also common in early onset PD, and it may also point toward a genetic form of the disease. The lack of overt bradykinesia and rigidity is common in early onset tremor-dominant PD. Subtle signs may be difficult to detect in older individuals. Mild reduced facial expression is often a subjective finding and cannot be reliably used to diagnose PD. A positive glabellar tap (repetitive nonrhythmical tapping between the eyebrows with the eyes open and asking the patient to try not to blink; it is positive when the patient continues to blink) can sometimes assist. The entity of so-called "benign tremulous PD" has been coined due to the milder clinical phenotype (thus little rigidity or bradykinesia) in these individuals, including a slower progression with much less motor disability as well as less risk of nonmotor symptoms such as mood and cognitive problems. Pathology in such individuals shows less severe nigral dopamine cell loss, which reflects this milder phenotype.

Essential tremor can cause leg tremor, but it would be bilateral and most likely associated with arm postural and intention tremor. Other causes of leg tremor include orthostatic tremor, which may be asymmetric but is bilateral and occurs after standing for a few seconds (delayed) and is also high frequency.

Dystonic tremor can also occur in the leg. Here, the primary abnormality is dystonia, and the tremor is secondary. In this individual, the foot and toe tremor is associated with the toe dystonia. Careful examination will help determine if the symptoms are related. Other causes of leg tremor with dystonia include metabolic disorders of catecholamine metabolism, especially dopamine, that cause dopa-responsive dystonia.

In this individual, genetic testing revealed a triphosphate cyclohydrolase-1 (*GCH-1*) gene mutation; thus, the final diagnosis was dopa-responsive dystonia (DRD). She was commenced on low-dose levodopa/carbidopa 100/25 mg 1 tab twice a day, with excellent improvement.

DOPA-RESPONSIVE DYSTONIA

Dopa-responsive dystonia (DRD) (DYT5) is commonly due to *GCH-1* mutations that lead to a disorder of dopamine metabolism with deficiency of tetrahydrobioptrin and subsequent abnormalities of biogenic amine synthesis. DRD is classically childhood-onset with dystonia starting in the legs and a diurnal variability such that children wake up with no or mild symptoms but have increased disability, particularly walking, toward the end of the day. The phenotype of DRD is expanding, and older individuals are increasingly recognized with delayed or variable onset of symptoms. The most common adult-onset clinical features involve focal dystonias and parkinsonism. The exact link between *GCH-1* mutations and PD remains unclear because families with rare *GCH-1* mutations have been described with young-onset typical DRD and older-onset PD associated with abnormal dopamine terminal scans.

Making a diagnosis of DRD in an adult typically involves a therapeutic trial of low-dose levodopa. Genetic testing may be useful to confirm DRD (although there are more than 200 mutations in the *GCH-1* gene) and rule out other causes of dystonia and tremor.

<table>
<tr><td>KEY POINTS TO REMEMBER</td></tr>
</table>

- Take time with the neurological examination to ensure you do not miss subtle dystonia.
- Remember that classic childhood-onset disorders can present in adults.
- Dystonic tremor may be a feature of several genetic dystonia syndromes, and a trial of levodopa may be warranted to ensure you do not miss late-onset DRD.

Further Reading

Balint B, Bhatia KP. Dystonia: An update on phenomenology, classification, pathogenesis and treatment. *Curr Opin Neurol* 2014;27(4):468–476.

Defazio G, Conte A, Gigante AF, Fabbrini G, Berardelli A. Is tremor in dystonia a phenotypic feature of dystonia? *Neurology* 2015;84(10):1053–1059.

Lewthwaite AJ, Lambert TD, Rolfe EB, et al. Novel GCH1 variant in dopa-responsive dystonia and Parkinson's disease. *Parkinsonism Relat Disord* 2015;21(4):394–397.

Mencacci NE, Isaias IU, Reich MM, et al.; International Parkinson's Disease Genomics Consortium and UCL-Exomes Consortium. Parkinson's disease in GTP cyclohydrolase 1 mutation carriers. *Brain* 2014;137(Pt 9):2480–2492.

Wijemanne S, Jankovic J. Dopa-responsive dystonia—Clinical and genetic heterogeneity. *Nat Rev Neurol* 2015 Jul;11(7):414–424.

28 A Rapidly Progressive Movement Disorder

Susan H. Fox and Marina Picillo

You see a 71-year-old right-handed woman with hypertension and dyslipidemia. She has a 2-month history of disorientation and gait and speech abnormalities, with progressive worsening and significant impact on her activities of daily living. She had no prior cognitive complaints and has no family history of neurological disease. She denies fever or any recent infection.

On examination she appears bradyphrenic with reduced verbal fluency and disorientation in time. She is hypomimic. There is mild bilateral upper limb rigidity and bradykinesia (left > right). With posture and action there are fine, irregular jerky movements of the fingers on both sides. Hand movements are dyspraxic with occasional left arm dystonic posturing and levitation. She has cortical sensory signs (astereognosia and agraphesthesia), especially on her left side. Her gait is wide-based, slow, and short-stepped, with spontaneous loss of balance when unsupported.

What do you do now?

MOVEMENT DISORDERS IN PRION DISEASE

When presented with any clinical syndrome such as this, first determine how the clinical signs fit together and what sort of underlying pathological process could contribute to such a rapidly progressive course. The combination of cortical findings (cognitive impairment, cortical sensory loss, dyspraxia, and myoclonus) and sub-cortical findings (parkinsonism, dystonia, and levitation) could be consistent with a rare clinical syndrome of multiple etiologies called corticobasal syndrome (CBS).

CBS can be seen as a consequence of a number of neurodegenerative etiologies, most commonly occurring in the seventh and eighth decades and seen in movement disorder clinics as a very asymmetrical parkinsonism with dystonia, myoclonus, and cortical signs affecting predominantly the upper limb. The underlying proteinopathy can be that of progressive supranuclear palsy, Alzheimer's disease, or corticobasal degeneration. However, a CBS with rapid onset and fast progression is strongly suggestive of a prion disease or Creutzfeldt–Jakob disease (CJD) (a list of the human transmissible prion diseases is provided in Box 28.1).

In general, the course of dementia in prion disease is rapidly progressive, generally of 2 years or less in duration, and with a rate of progression much faster than in more common neurodegenerative diseases. The onset is typically subacute (i.e., days to weeks), in contrast to other disorders, in which an exact date of onset is often difficult to identify. Focal higher cortical signs are typical (aphasia, acalculia, neglect, and apraxia). Astereognosis can be tested by asking the patient to close his or her eyes and identify an object placed in the patient's hands. Dysgraphesthesia is sought by tracing letters or numbers onto the palm of either hand, respectively. Behavioral features are common first symptoms and may include psychotic symptoms, depression, and personality changes. When evaluating a patient with a subacute onset of movement disorder with dementia, a specific list of conditions should be considered in the differential diagnosis (Table 28.1), particularly those that are treatable.

BOX 28.1 **Human Prion Diseases or Transmissible Spongiform Encephalopathies**

1. Creutzfeldt–Jacob disease (CJD)
   Sporadic (sCJD)
   Iatrogenic
   New variant (vCJD)
   Familial
2. Gerstmann–Sträussler–Scheinker disease (GSS)
3. Fatal familial insomnia (FFI)
4. Kuru

TABLE 28.1 **Possible Causes of Rapid-Onset Movement Disorders with Dementia**

Vascular	• Multiple infarcts • Cerebral amyloid angiopathy • Vasculitis/angiitis
Infectious	• Encephalitis (bacterial, viral, fungal) • HIV/AIDS • Syphilis • Lyme disease • Whipple's disease • Progressive multifocal leukoencephalopathy • Subacute sclerosis panencephalitis
Toxic-metabolic	• Vitamin deficiency (B_6, niacin, thiamin) • Bismuth encephalopathy • Wilson's disease • Porphyria
Autoimmune	• Anti-NMDA encephalopathy • VGKC-associated encephalopathy • Anti-GAD encephalopathy • Hashimoto encephalopathy • Behçet's disease • Sarcoidosis
Metastatic/Cancer	• Infiltrating tumors • Lymphoma • Paraneoplastic encephalopathy (e.g., anti-Hu, VGKC, NMDA)
Iatrogenic	• Medications
Neurodegenerative	• Prion disease • Rapidly progressive diffuse Lewy body disease • Frontotemporal lobar degeneration with/without motor neuron disease • Tauopathies (progressive supranuclear palsy, corticobasal degeneration) • Alzheimer's disease
Systemic	• Mitochondrial

GAD, glutamic acid decarboxylase; NMDA, N-methyl-D-aspartate; VGKC, voltage-gated potassium channel.
Source: Adapted from Geschwind MD. Rapidly progressive dementia: Prion diseases and other rapid dementias. *Continuum (Minneap Minn)* 2010;16(2):31–56.

INVESTIGATIONS

The next step is to perform investigations to try to determine the cause of the CBS, including an electroencephalogram (EEG), cerebrospinal fluid (CSF) examination, and magnetic resonance imaging (MRI) of the brain. Whereas diffuse slowing and frontal rhythmic delta activity are rather nonspecific, periodic or pseudo-periodic sharp-wave complexes are typical EEG findings in middle/late-stage sporadic CJD (sCJD) (Fig. 28.1A). CSF testing is mandatory to rule out infectious etiologies, but it can also be helpful to suggest a neurodegenerative origin if biomarker studies are available. The 14-3-3 protein is the most reliable among several CSF diagnostic markers for prion diseases, although the specificity is poor. The overall reported sensitivity of the Western blot test for the 14-3-3 protein in sCJD is 85–97%, whereas specificity has been reported to range between 28% and 97%. Real-time quaking-induced conversion is a new technique highly specific for detecting abnormal prion protein and, according to recent data, might be more sensitive when using olfactory epithelium (from nasal brushings) than CSF.

Brain MRI is fundamental for the diagnosis of vascular and cancer causes, and it may also be helpful in supporting an alternative neurodegenerative entity. Recently, cerebral cortical signal increase and high signal in caudate nucleus and putamen on fluid attenuated inversion recovery (FLAIR) or diffusion-weighted

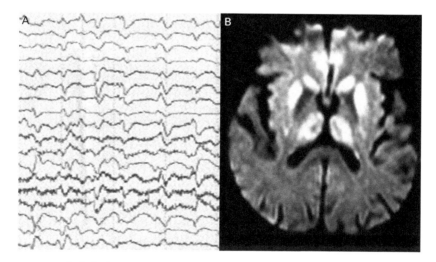

FIGURE 28.1 Periodic sharp-wave complex occurring every 1–3 seconds (A) and DWI MRI showing decreased diffusivity in the basal ganglia and thalamus (B).

Source: Reprinted with permission from Kallenberg K, Schulz-Schaeffer WJ, Jastrow U, et al. Creutzfeldt–Jakob disease: Comparative analysis of MR imaging sequences. Am J Neuroradiol 2006;27(7):1459–1462.

imaging (DWI) MRI (Fig. 28.1B) were reported to be a useful addiction for the diagnosis of sCJD (Box 28.2).

PRION DISEASES

Prion diseases are transmissible, progressive, and invariably fatal neurodegenerative conditions associated with misfolding and aggregation of a host-encoded cellular prion protein, PrPC. The most common form of human prion disease is sCJD, with an incidence of approximately 1 case per 1 million persons per year worldwide and a typical age of onset between 55 and 75 years. Possible or probable sCJD is defined on the basis of clinical features as well as results of specific investigations (i.e., EEG, CSF testing, and brain MRI). Diagnostic criteria for sCJD are displayed in Box 28.2. Definite diagnosis requires neuropathological or immunochemical detection of the prion protein in brain tissue. Iatrogenic CJD has been related to corneal graft transplantation, contaminated human pituitary-derived growth hormone or gonadotropin, and dura mater grafts. The rare new variant CJD (vCJD) is related to bovine spongiform encephalopathy, with more than 200 vCJD cases reported since 1996, the majority in the United Kingdom. A younger age of onset (mid-teens to early 40s) characterizes vCJD, along with a relatively longer illness duration (range, 4–25 months). Clinical features are often limited to psychiatric disturbance or sensory symptoms, until ataxia, cognitive impairment, and involuntary movements develop later in the course.

Genetic or familial forms of prion diseases are due to autosomal dominant mutations in the PRNP gene encoding the prion protein and include familial CJD, Gerstmann–Sträussler–Scheinker disease (GSS), and fatal familial insomnia (FFI). GSS mainly occurs between 40 and 60 years of age and is characterized by cerebellar dysfunction, gait disturbance, dementia, and mild dysarthria with considerable intrafamilial and intragenerational variability. FFI presents between 20 and 72 years of age and is caused by a PRNP mutation *D178N* linked to methionine of the PRNP polymorphism M129V. It is clinically characterized by a profound disruption of the normal sleep–wake cycle with complete disorganization of the EEG patterns of sleep (agrypnia excitata), associated with autonomic hyperactivity and somatomotor abnormalities (pyramidal signs, myoclonus, dysarthria/dysphagia, and gait dysfunctions). Polysomnographic recording is helpful in the diagnosis of FFI. PRNP genetic testing is mandatory for confirmation of familial forms of prion diseases.

MYOCLONUS AND OTHER MOVEMENT DISORDERS IN PRION DISEASE

The prevalence of movement disorders in patients with prion diseases is high, occurring in approximately 90% of patients during the disease course. Myoclonus is by far the most common movement disorder associated with all CJD variants as well as with FFI, whereas it is less frequent in GSS. Focal or generalized jerks have been reported to occur in 82–100% of CJD cases during the course of the disease, no matter the genotype. Myoclonic jerks are often diffuse, generalized, relatively rhythmic, and associated with periodic sharp-wave EEG activity. They are emphasized by noise and/or sensitive stimuli (startle myoclonus) and can also be associated with other movement disorders, such as athetoid movements of the fingers, alien hand, or dystonic posturing. In these cases, myoclonus jerks are frequently asymmetric, affecting the distal extremity of limbs, and can occur early within the course of the disease. Generalized dystonia has been more commonly reported at the later stage of the disease and is usually preceded by focal dystonia that has progressively worsened. Chorea is a common later stage symptom in vCJD and is often superimposed on a variety of involuntary movements, such as dystonic postures. Concerning gait disorders, ataxia is by far the most common, being present in up to 84% of patients with CJD. Extrapyramidal syndromes (especially akinetic mutism) are a classical feature of the terminal stages of prion diseases. However, parkinsonism may occur as an initial presentation of CJD in the form of CBS or accompanied by vertical gaze limitation, thus mimicking a progressive supranuclear palsy. Tremor is commonly associated with dystonic postures, and its differentiation from myoclonic jerks is often challenging.

Beyond the cognitive impairment, GSS is characterized by cerebellar symptoms, including gait unsteadiness, limb ataxia with dysmetria, dysdiadochokinesis, and intention tremor. In addition, there may be signs of corticospinal tract degeneration, such as limb weakness, spasticity, hyperreflexia, and extensor plantar responses. Some families with GSS (especially those carrying the codon 105 proline-to-leucine mutation, *P105L*) may present spastic paraparesis alone in the absence of any cerebellar symptoms.

Although FFI is dominated by sleep disorder and dysautonomia, as the disease progresses, a range of motor abnormalities usually evolve in variable combinations with cerebellar and pyramidal dysfunctions culminating in prominent limb, gait, and bulbar difficulties. Cognitive decline and dementia usually appear in late stages.

MANAGEMENT

Although several compounds have been tested in recent years, prion diseases remain fatal encephalopathies with no effective treatment available. Mean survival is between 4 and 8 months, with 90% of patients with CJD dying within 1 year and within 18.4 months for those with FFI. GSS demonstrates slower disease progression over a period of 3½–9½ years. Due to its unconventional transmission and invariable fatality, CJD poses a serious risk to public health. Physicians caring for patients with suspect prion disease should be aware of national surveillance protocols (World Health Organization).

KEY POINTS TO REMEMBER

- Movement disorders represent a prominent feature of prion diseases and include cerebellar and extrapyramidal symptoms. Myoclonus is by far the most common involuntary movement in prion diseases.
- Suspicion of a prion disease in the presence of a rapidly progressive dementia is mandatory.
- Diagnosis is based on clinical features and results of investigations (EEG, CSF testing, and brain MRI). PRNP genetic analysis is mandatory in familial forms.
- Prion diseases are fatal encephalopathies with no effective treatment available. Due to the unconventional transmission mechanism, prion diseases represent a serious risk to public health. Awareness of national surveillance protocols is necessary when dealing with such patients.

Further Reading

Cortelli P, Fabbri M, Calandra-Buonaura G, et al. Gait disorders in fatal familial insomnia. *Mov Disord* 2014;29(3):420–424.

Edler J, Mollenhauer B, Heinemann U, et al. Movement disturbances in the differential diagnosis of Creutzfeldt–Jakob disease. *Mov Disord* 2008;24(3):350–356.

Imran M, Mahmood S. An overview of human prion diseases. *Virol J* 2011 24;8:559.

Maltete D, Guyant-Marechal L, Mihout B, Hannequin D. Movement disorders and Creutzfeldt–Jakob disease: A review. *Parkinsonism Relat Disord* 2006;12:65–71.

Zeidler M, Gibbs CJ, Meslin F. WHO manual for strengthening diagnosis and surveillance of Creutzfeldt–Jakob disease (WHO/EMC/ZDI/98.11). Geneva: World Health Organization, 1998.

Zerr I, Kallenberg K, Summers DM, et al. Updated clinical diagnostic criteria for sporadic Creutzfeldt–Jakob disease. *Brain* 2009;132(Pt 10):2659–2668.

PART VI

Movement Disorder Emergencies

29 Wakeful Unresponsiveness

Susan H. Fox

A 26-year-old woman presented to the emergency room
with a 3-week history of "bizarre" behaviors—she was
intermittently disorientated and confused. She would not
sleep at night but during the day appeared drowsy and at
times unrousable. She had complained of headaches and
did not like bright lights. The emergency room physicians
are concerned about meningitis, and they immediately
started her on appropriate intravenous broad-spectrum
antibiotics. While preparing her for the lumbar puncture
they notice she has abnormal random movements in
her face and arms, and they are struggling to keep her
still due to agitation and movements. They call for a
neurology consultation.

What do you do now?

ANTI-NMDA RECEPTOR ENCEPHALITIS

Define the Phenomenology

More history needs to be obtained from the family. The term "confusion" needs to be explored because it can mean different things to different people, from an isolated speech disturbance to a complex partial seizure. Further questioning of family reveals that the patient has had visual and auditory hallucinations, culminating in the past 2 weeks to increasing paranoia and inability to sleep at night. She had been forgetful and at times her speech was bizarre and inappropriate. The family had noticed some abnormal chewing movements. There was no known history of drug abuse, and she was not taking any prescribed medications. She had no relevant prior medical history. Two months ago, she vacationed in the Caribbean but did not report any problems. On your examination, she is febrile (temperature 38°C). She has low blood pressure (90/50). She is intermittently agitated and restless. She has orofacial chorea. The remainder of the neurological examination appears normal.

What Do You Do Next?

Determining the cause of orofacial movements in a young woman depends on the history and other associated clinical findings (Box 29.1). She has a mixture of psychosis and behavioral changes combined with orofacial chorea. Acute psychosis in a young woman may indicate the start of a primary psychiatric disorder such as schizophrenia; however, the associated neurological symptoms would make a secondary cause more likely. The most likely clinical diagnosis is encephalitis. The causes of encephalitis include infective and noninfective etiologies (Box 29.2).

The initial investigations should include blood and urinalysis and urgent cerebrospinal fluid (CSF) for protein, glucose, and cell count, in addition to polymerase chain reaction (PCR) for herpes and varicella viruses with culture and sensitivity to determine if there is an infectious cause. The CSF should also be sent for autoantibody screen because there is evidence that intrathecal autoantibody production has a greater specificity in autoantibody-mediated encephalopathies. The presence of a fever does not always indicate an infection, and up to 50% of autoimmune encephalitis can also cause fever and some autonomic dysfunction. Prodromal symptoms such as headache also occur in noninfectious encephalitis. Antibiotics or antivirals, however, should always be commenced, if appropriate, while waiting for test results. An untreated viral encephalitis is a far greater risk than a period of unnecessary acyclovir pending viral PCR results. Brain imaging in encephalitis can be useful, although it is not

BOX 29.1 **Differential Diagnosis of Acute Orofacial Involuntary Movements in a Young Woman**

Seizure-related movements
    Status epilepticus
Chorea
    Drugs
        Stimulants (cocaine, amphetamine, PCP)
        Oral contraceptive pill
    Paroxysmal kinesiogenic dyskinesia
Dystonia
    Following initiation of antipsychotic
Combined with other neurological findings
    Encephalitis (see Box 29.2)
        Infectious (e.g., viral)
        Noninfectious—for example, autoimmune (e.g., thyroid, lupus
            antibody, postpartum)
    Neuroleptic malignant syndrome
    Stroke
    Metabolic dysfunction (glucose, renal, liver, thyroid)
    Wilson's disease
    Demyelination (acute disseminated encephalomyelitis, multiple
        sclerosis)

always diagnostic and is often normal. Herpes simplex encephalitis may show asymmetrical medial temporal changes, but autoimmune encephalitis can also show increased T2 signal in medial temporal lobes and nonspecific fluid attenuated inversion recovery (FLAIR) changes in cortical regions.

BOX 29.2 **Causes of Acute Encephalitis**

Infectious—herpes simplex encephalitis, varicella zoster
Metabolic—renal, liver
Autoimmune
    Thyroid—lupus antibody-mediated
    Paraneoplastic antibody-mediated associated with lung, thymus,
        breast, testicular cancers
    Anti-Hu, -CRMP5, -Ri, -Ma2, -GAD65, -Yo—most common association
        with tumors
    Amphiphysin, GAD65—stiff person syndrome
    NMDAR, GABAbR, AMPA, mGlur5, LGI1, CASPR2, DPPX—less
        common association with cancer

The patient's initial blood and urinalysis were negative. CSF revealed normal protein and glucose but a slightly elevated lymphocyte count. Brain magnetic resonance imaging was normal.

How Are You Going to Treat Her?

The patient was already on antibiotics and acyclovir by emergency room staff, and you continue these for the first 48 hours. However, she does not improve, and she still has involuntary facial movements. She was commenced on intravenous immunoglobulin. Early treatment with immunotherapy can improve outcomes and should be started as soon as possible if the index of suspicion is high for an autoimmune encephalitis (as in this case); this should not wait for antibody testing.

Autoantibody testing in blood and CSF was positive for the GluNR1 subunit of the NMDR receptor. A computed tomography scan of her abdomen and pelvis revealed an ovarian teratoma. Surgical resection resulted in a full recovery.

NMDA RECEPTOR ENCEPHALITIS DEFINED

This is one of the most common forms of autoimmune encephalitis in young people. Presentation is usually in young women (average age, 20 years) and is commonly associated with ovarian teratomas. Clinically, patients present with neuropsychiatric symptoms and associated dyskinesia (especially orofacial) and in some cases seizures. Autonomic instability can also occur. In some individuals, acute psychiatric symptoms including hallucinations, delusions, or mania can be the initial presentation, and young persons may be misdiagnosed as having schizophrenia.

The antibody is against the NR1a subunit of the NMDA receptor. Rarer antibodies against different antigens (e.g., the NR2a and NR2b subunits) have been described. Enhanced glutamate receptor activation is responsible for the phenotype of psychosis and hyperkinetic movements. Recognition and early appropriate treatment is important. Three-fourths of patients can recover, although this can take several months. Recovery is better if immunotherapy (corticosteroids, intravenous immunoglobulins, or plasma exchange) is started within the first 4 weeks of the disease and additional surgical removal of any identified teratomas. Second-line immunotherapy includes rituximab or cyclophosphamide. There is a risk of relapse in some individuals. A worse outcome or risk of relapse is correlated to higher levels of NMDA receptor antibody in CSF and serum.

- Always search for secondary causes of acute-onset psychosis in a young person.
- Orofacial chorea is a common symptom associated with autoimmune encephalitis due to anti-NMAD receptor antibodies.
- Immunotherapy should be started early in patients with noninfectious encephalitis because antibody testing may be delayed or negative.

Further Reading

Barry H, Byrne S, Barrett E, Murphy KC, Cotter DR. Anti-*N*-methyl-d-aspartate receptor encephalitis: Review of clinical presentation, diagnosis and treatment. *BJPsych Bull* 2015 Feb;39(1):19–23.

Kayser MS, Titulaer MJ, Gresa-Arribas N, Dalmau J. Frequency and characteristics of isolated psychiatric episodes in anti-*N*-methyl-d-aspartate receptor encephalitis. *JAMA Neurol* 2013 Sep 1;70(9):1133–1139.

Titulaer MJ, McCracken L, Gabilondo I, et al. Treatment and prognostic factors for long-term outcome in patients with anti-NMDA receptor encephalitis: An observational cohort study. *Lancet Neurol* 2013;12(2):157–165.

30 An Iatrogenic Catatonia

Robertus M. A. de Bie

The patient is a 35-year-old male alcoholic who stopped drinking alcohol 4 days ago. He developed symptoms of an alcohol withdrawal syndrome. Subsequently, the family physician treated him with chlordiazepoxide 100 mg BID and haloperidol 5 mg/day. He started to experience stiffness of his legs, which progressively worsened, and he was unable to eat. Altogether, he was given haloperidol 5 mg on two occasions. At the emergency unit, he was alert. His blood pressure was 100/70 mm Hg, the heart rate was 100 beats per minute, and his temperature was 38.3°C. He had dysarthria, a stiff neck, orofacial dyskinesias, and hypertonic arms and legs. A lumbar puncture was performed with normal findings. Plasma sodium, creatinine, and the leukocyte concentration were normal. The erythrocyte sedimentation rate was 30 mm, and the creatine phosphokinase (CPK) level was elevated up to 20 times the upper limit of normal.

What do you do now?

TABLE 30.1 **Manifestations of NMS, Serotonin Syndrome, and Anticholinergic Poisoning**

Condition	Medication History	Time Needed for Condition to Develop	Vital Signs	Pupils	Mucosa	Skin	Bowel Sounds	Muscle Tone	Reflexes	Mental Status
NMS	Dopamine antagonist	1–3 days	Hypertension, tachycardia, tachypnea, hyperthermia (>41.1°C)	Normal	Sialorrhea	Pallor, diaphoresis	Normal or decreased	"Lead-pipe" rigidity present in all muscle groups	Normal	Fluctuating consciousness, from being alert to coma
Serotonin syndrome	Two or three serotonergic drugs at the same time	<12 hours	Hypertension, tachycardia, tachypnea, hyperthermia (>41.1°C)	Mydriasis	Sialorrhea	Diaphoresis	Hyperactive	Increased, predominantly in lower extremities	Hyperreflexia, clonus	Agitated, coma
Anticholinergic poisoning	Anticholinergic agent	<12 hours	Hypertension (mild), tachycardia, tachypnea, hyperthermia (typically 38.8°C or less)	Mydriasis	Dry	Erythema, hot and dry to touch	Decreased or absent	Normal	Normal	Agitated, delirium

NEUROLEPTIC MALIGNANT SYNDROME

This patient has a neuroleptic malignant syndrome (NMS) in addition to an alcohol withdrawal syndrome. The incidence of NMS is between 0.007% and 0.9% of admitted patients who use a neuroleptic drug. NMS can occur at all ages and is twice as frequent in men compared to women. All neuroleptics can cause NMS, including the newer atypical antipsychotics. Possible risk factors for NMS are dehydration and an earlier episode of NMS. There seems to be no relationship with the dose of the offending drug. The exact pathophysiological mechanism is not known, although the abrupt dopamine blockade appears to be an important contributing factor for the development of NMS.

The clinical picture may consist of a relatively slow onset, with fever, muscle stiffness, fluctuating consciousness, and autonomic instability. The CPK is often elevated due to muscle injury and can be used to monitor the disease course; a decreasing CPK with an increasing temperature may indicate an infection. In addition, leukocytosis may occur. If the neuroleptic is stopped, the signs and symptoms may persist for 2–14 days. Mortality is 10%. The differential diagnosis includes the serotonin syndrome, anticholinergic poisoning, and malignant hyperthermia, each of which can be distinguished from NMS on clinical grounds and the medication history (Table 30.1).

The most important act is to stop the neuroleptic drug. Further treatment involves providing supportive care: lowering the temperature with antipyretics and cold blankets; administering intravenous fluids; preventing deep vein thrombosis; and, if necessary, correcting the electrolyte disorders, giving antihypertensives, and providing extra oxygen. Pharmacological therapies may be tried, although they are not proven effective. These are bromocriptine (2.5 mg TID) and dantrolene (intravenous bolus of 1–10 mg/kg followed by a maintenance dose of 600 mg/day).

In this case, we started intravenous dantrolene 70 mg QID, thiamine 100 mg/day, extra intravenous fluids, and diazepam. The following day, temperature and muscle tone were normalized. A couple of days later, he developed a pneumonia, which was treated successfully with antibiotics.

KEY POINTS TO REMEMBER

- The most important therapy of NMS is to stop the neuroleptic.
- All neuroleptics can produce NMS, including the new atypical antipsychotics.
- CPK can be used to monitor the disease course; a decreasing CPK with an increasing temperature may indicate an infection.

Further Reading

Boyer EW, Shannon M. The serotonin syndrome. *N Engl J Med* 2005;352:1112–1120.

Guze BH, Baxter LRJr. Neuroleptic malignant syndrome. *N Engl J Med* 1985;313:163–166.

Pelonero AL, Levenson JL, Pandurangi AK. Neuroleptic malignant syndrome: A review. *Psych Ser* 1998;49:1163–1172.

31 Always Worth a Second Look

Richard A. Walsh

You are called to the surgical ward by a colleague to give an opinion on a 77-year-old woman who has returned from theater following an elective hemiarthroplasty. She has a history of depression and diabetes mellitus. She is conscious but agitated upon your arrival on the ward. Her perioperative course had been uneventful initially. In the recovery room, she had recovered well and had been able to speak to the nursing staff. Intramuscular tramadol had been administered to relieve postoperative pain on return to the ward. The staff became concerned when her level of consciousness deteriorated with confused speech and what are described as jerks involving her lower limbs predominantly.

On examination she has a temperature of 38°C/100.4°F and a tachycardia of 110. There are intermittent myoclonic jerks, and she appears generally tremulous. She will not answer any questions or obey commands. Tone appears increased in both lower limbs with brisk knee and ankle jerks and spontaneous clonus at the ankles bilaterally. Plantar responses are extensor.

What do you do now?

SEROTONIN SYNDROME

Serotonin syndrome is one of a group of acute iatrogenic syndromes with shared clinical features, which include altered consciousness, autonomic dysregulation, and features of neuromuscular irritability. Although often considered together, serotonin syndrome, neuroleptic malignant syndrome, and the Parkinson's hyperpyrexia syndrome can be distinguished on the basis of particular clinical clues and a thorough drug history. An appropriate level of suspicion is required, and as with many rarer conditions, it is only when you experience your first case that you will begin to consider and recognize it more often. There are undoubtedly many *forms frustes* of serotonin syndrome, on the lower end of the spectrum of toxicity, which hospital physicians may pass by unknowingly on a regular basis. An awareness of vulnerable groups of patients is helpful. These include patients on psychiatric drugs, particularly with polypharmacy; patients being treated for Parkinson's disease; and patients in the perioperative setting, in which analgesic agents and fentanyl are commonly used. Always take a second look at the list of drugs being administered.

Pathophysiology

Less than 10% of serotonin synthesis is central, with the remainder being located in the periphery, and predominantly the gastrointestinal tract where it is prokinetic. The serotonin syndrome is a drug toxicity syndrome, attributed to excessive postsynaptic serotoninergic receptor stimulation at 5-HT1A and 5-HT2A receptors. This syndrome has classically been associated with nonselective monoamine oxidase inhibitor (MAOI) antidepressant use in conjunction with other serotonergic agents—a combination often resulting in the most severe cases. With the move away from these agents, the selective serotonin reuptake inhibitors (SSRIs) and serotonin noradrenaline reuptake inhibitors (SNRIs) are now more commonly implicated given their widespread use. In most cases, it is a combination of two or more agents that is the cause, through either stimulation of serotonin release, inhibition of its metabolism, or exertion of a serotoninergic effect at a receptor level. Serotonin syndrome is unusual with serotoninergic monotherapy, occurring in only 14–16% of patients following an SSRI overdose. Spending time on a recent drug history is critical, both prescribed and recreational, particularly with respect to recent changes because serotonin syndrome will typically manifest within 24 hours of a new drug or a dose increase (Table 31.1).

Individual susceptibility arising from genetically determined activity of the MAO enzyme may be an important inherited risk factor for serotonin syndrome.

TABLE 31.1 **Drug Classes Associated with Serotonin Toxicity and Proposed Mechanism**

Class	Agents	Proposed Mechanism
Antidepressants	SSRI and SNRIs	↓ reuptake
	Nonselective MAOIs	↓ MAO metabolism
	TCAs	↓ MAO metabolism
	Trazadone	↓ MAO metabolism
	Lithium	↓ reuptake
Pain medications	Fentanyl	↓ reuptake
	Tramadol	↓ reuptake
	Triptans	5-HT receptor agonist
Antimicrobials	Linezolid	↓ MAO metabolism
Antiparkinsonian drugs	Selegiline and rasagiline	↓ MAO metabolism
	Levodopa	↓ reuptake
	Dopamine agonists	↓ reuptake
	Amantadine	↓ reuptake
Recreational drugs	Amphetamines	↑ release
	Cocaine	↑ release
Others	St. John's wort	↓ reuptake
	Methylene blue	

MAOI, monoamine oxidase inhibitor; SNRI, serotonin noradrenaline reuptake inhibitor; SSRI, selective serotonin reuptake inhibitor; TCA, tricyclic antidepressant.

Acquired variability of serotonin metabolism arising from smoking, chronic liver disease, and pulmonary disease are additional risk factors.

Clinical Features

The clinical features of serotonin syndrome can be divided broadly into three categories, each of which can manifest in varying severity. Alterations of consciousness through a direct toxic effect of serotonin on the central nervous system (CNS) can lead to mild changes such as irritability, agitation, hypervigilance, and hypomania or in more severe cases can give rise to a frank delirium or coma. Autonomic instability can consist of diaphoresis, mydriasis, tachycardia, and hyperthermia. Gastrointestinal disturbance (diarrhea and increased bowel sounds) can also be observed. Neuromuscular irritability is characterized by clonus (spontaneous or inducible) and hyperreflexia, often prominent in the lower limbs; myoclonus; tremor; and increased muscle tone. Creatine kinase (CK) may be elevated in more severe cases. See Box 31.1 for the Hunter serotonin toxicity criteria.

Differential Diagnosis

Neuroleptic Malignant Syndrome

Neuroleptic malignant syndrome (NMS) is typically slower in onset, over days not hours. The conscious patient with serotonin syndrome can be found babbling incoherently, whereas NMS is characterized by an akinetic rigid state without speech output. In NMS, the tone increase is generalized and extrapyramidal, whereas in serotonin syndrome it is lower limb predominant and pyramidal with associated pyramidal features.

Parkinson's Hyperpyrexia Syndrome

Parkinson's hyperpyrexia syndrome can mimic serotonin syndrome, but it has greater clinical similarity and shared pathophysiology with neuroleptic malignant syndrome. Both are syndromes of frontal subcortical dopaminergic depletion, although in the case of Parkinson's hyperpyrexia syndrome it is a withdrawal of dopaminergic medication that gives rise to the observed clinical features rather than administration of drugs with D2 receptor antagonism. Recovery is typically more prolonged and mortality greater in this group of vulnerable patients. It is worth noting that introduction of levodopa has been independently linked with serotonin syndrome.

Of further relevance in patients with Parkinson's disease is the strong and traditional association between the MAOI drug class and serotonin syndrome, often leading to concern when the MAO-B inhibitors selegiline and rasagiline are co-prescribed with SSRIs or SNRIs. Soon after patients leave the clinic, pharmacies will typically call to question the safety of this combination. The incidence of serotonin in this scenario is very small compared with the risk of a similar combination with nonselective MAO inhibitors with SSRIs (up to 50%).

Alcohol Withdrawal

The delirium tremens following alcohol withdrawal will present with a confusional state, general tremulousness, agitation, and a tachycardia. Serum CK may be raised in a patient who has been lying on the ground in an alcohol-related stupor. Furthermore, acute alcohol withdrawal can be associated with parkinsonism that is typically mild and fully reversible. The mechanism of this transient parkinsonism is poorly understood. The overall picture of recent significant alcohol consumption should be readily apparent. Administration of neuroleptics, as sometimes employed in acute alcohol withdrawal states, to a patient with NMS is to be avoided.

Cholinergic or Opioid Toxicity

Alternative toxic syndromes warrant consideration if the drug history does not fit with a serotonin syndrome. Rapid escalation in opioid dose can give rise to a hyperexcitability syndrome. Unlike many other opioids, morphine does not inhibit serotonin reuptake, but it is metabolized to morphine-3-glucuronide, which can be associated with a hyperexcitability syndrome. Cholinergic toxicity can cause a delirium, but the bowel involvement is the opposite with constipation, and reduced bowel sounds and pupillary changes are meiotic, not mydriatic. Small pupil size is seen with cholinergic toxicity as opposed to mydriasis in serotonin syndrome.

CNS Infective States (e.g., a Meningoencephalitis)

Meningitis can look similar to serotonin syndrome, with prominent axial rigidity, pyrexia, tachycardia, and pyramidal signs in the limbs. These patients will have features of sepsis such as raised inflammatory markers, and there may be a helpful collateral history of a prodromal headache and photophobia, which would not fit with a serotonin syndrome. If there is any doubt and in particular where there is no recent drug history, a low threshold for performing a lumbar puncture is required and routine cerebrospinal fluid analysis will discriminate between infective and noninfective states.

Management

Withdrawal of the offending agent is typically sufficient to produce a reasonably quick turnaround in most mild to moderate cases. Supportive care is the mainstay of management, with an emphasis on ensuring adequate hydration and monitoring renal indices and for urinary myoglobin when CK is markedly raised. Use of thromboprophylaxis with subcutaneous low-molecular-weight heparin is advisable until normal mobility is resumed. Only the most severe cases will require admission to an intensive care unit, and this may be for monitoring of autonomic instability, ventilation, and dialysis when renal failure complicates rhabdomyolysis. Failure to settle within 24–48 hours of discontinuation of the responsible agent(s) should prompt a reconsideration of the diagnosis.

Drug therapy with benzodiazepines can settle agitation and help to normalize blood pressure and pulse rate. The antihistamine cyproheptadine has 5-HT1A and 5-HT2A antagonistic properties and is available only in tablet or syrup form for enteric administration to be given in a loading dose of 12 mg daily and maintenance of 4–8 mg every 6 hours for severe cases. There is little evidence for the use of cyproheptadine, although short-term use in the absence of significant side effects other than useful sedation makes it a reasonable option in more difficult cases.

In this case, the priority is recognition of multiple drug exposures that have precipitated serotonin syndrome to allow withdrawal and appropriate supportive care.

KEY POINTS TO REMEMBER

- Serotonin syndrome is a potentially life-threatening iatrogenic toxic state caused by excessive serotoninergic stimulation within the central nervous system.
- Serotonin syndrome is best considered a clinical spectrum rather than an all-or-nothing syndromic diagnosis. Misidentification of milder forms in hospitalized patients as a delirium is undoubtedly a common error.
- Fluoxetine, although a less potent serotoninergic drug, has a metabolite norfluoxetine with a half-life of up to 2 weeks, which can lead to serotonin toxicity when replaced with an alternative serotoninergic agent without an appropriate washout period.
- A key discriminating factor from neuroleptic malignant syndrome is the brief latency to onset after initiating or increase in serotoninergic drug and the rapid offset after discontinuation.

- Withdrawal of the drug(s) believed to be responsible and supportive care are the primary therapeutic steps.

Further Reading

Adler AR, Charnin JA, Quraishi SA. Serotonin syndrome: The potential for a severe reaction between common perioperative medications and selective serotonin reuptake inhibitors. *A A Case Rep.* 2015 Nov 1;5(9):156–159.

Buckley NA, Dawson AH, Isbister GK. Serotonin syndrome. *BMJ* 2014;348:g1626.

Graudins A, Stearman A, Chan B. Treatment of the serotonin syndrome with cyproheptadine. *J Emerg Med* 1998 Jul–Aug;16(4):615–619.

Perry PJ, Wilborn CA. Serotonin syndrome vs neuroleptic malignant syndrome: A contrast of causes, diagnoses, and management. *Ann Clin Psychiatry* 2012 May;24(2):155–162. [Review]

Index

Page numbers followed by *f*, *t*, and *b* indicates figures, tables, and boxes respectively.

management of, 91–92

parkinsonism with, 89

in patient with late-onset psychosis and
cognitive impairment, 55

depression

cognitive abilities affected by, 16

in PD, 25

palliative measures for, 37*t*

*Diagnostic and Statistical Manual of Mental
Disorders*, 5th ed. (DSM-5)

on functional movement
disorders, 181

diffuse cerebrovascular disease

gait apraxia due to, 108

distractibility

in functional movement disorders,
178*b*, 179

DJ1 (PARK7) mutations

monogenic PD and, 45*t*, 47

DLB. *see* dementia with Lewy
bodies (DLB)

donepezil

for cognitive impairment in PD, 19*t*

for DLB, 91

dopamine agonists

for PD, 4, 6, 7*t*

dopamine D2 antagonists

neurological side effects of, 158–159

"dopamine dysregulation syndrome," 12

dopaminergic therapies

for PD, 36

dopamine transporter (DaT) scan

in PD diagnosis, 52, 53*f*, 53*t*

indications for, 54–55

urgency in ordering, 52–53

dopa-responsive dystonia (DRD), 138, 197,
201–202

DRD. *see* dopa-responsive dystonia (DRD)

D2 receptor antagonist

in parkinsonism management

nigrostriatal system imaging in, 54

driving

by PD patients

criteria for, 20

drooling. *see* sialorrhea

drug(s)

choreas due to, 170*b*, 171

DSM-5. *see Diagnostic and Statistical Manual
of Mental Disorders*, 5th ed. (DSM-5)

DT. *see* dystonic tremor (DT)

dysarthria

hyperkinetic, 168

pseudobulbar

in PSP, 74

dysautonomia

in MSA, 62

management of, 65–66

dysgraphesthesia

testing of, 204

dyskinesia(s)

exercise-induced

seizures in, 132*t*

facial

in MSA, 63

functional paroxysmal, 197

levodopa and, 4

in MSA, 63

paroxysmal

classification of, 194–196

primary, 194

paroxysmal exercise-induced, 193–198

(*see also* paroxysmal exercise-induced
dyskinesia (PED))

paroxysmal kinesigenic (*see* paroxysmal
kinesigenic dyskinesia (PKD))

paroxysmal nonkinesigenic, 194, 195*t*, 196

tardive, 157–160 (*see also* tardive
dyskinesia)

dysphagia

in PD

indications for, 38*t*

sialorrhea and, 26

dysphasia

in CBS, 82

dyspraxia

defined, 80

ideational, 80–81

ideomotor, 80

in PSP, 74

types of, 80–81

dystonia(s), 127–154. *see also specific types, e.g.,*
Wilson's disease (WD)

acquired

DBS for, 146

tetrabenazine
  for tardive dystonia, 159
thyroiditis
  autoimmune
    steroid-responsive encephalopathy
      associated with, 97
tics
  described, 168
  focal dystonia *vs.*, 151
  tardive, 158
tongue tremor
  in MSA, 102
tonic spasms
  in MS, 197
Toronto Western Spasmodic
      Torticollis Rating Scale (TWSTRS),
      145, 146
torticollis
  spasmodic, 149
tracheostomy
  in MSA management, 62, 66
transcutaneous electrical nerve stimulation
      for DT, 138
transmissible spongiform encephalopathies
  types of, 204*b*
tremor(s). *see also specific types*
  with abnormal posture, 135–139 (*see also*
      dystonic tremor (DT))
  atypical
    in MSA, 62
  characteristics of
    in differential diagnosis, 162
  in CJD, 209
  described, 162–163, 162*b*
  with dystonia
    in adult, 200, 201*b*
  dystonia–gene associated, 136
  dystonic, 135–139 (*see also* dystonic
      tremor (DT))
  essential (*see* essential tremor)
  frequency of, 163
  in functional movement disorders,
      177–180, 177*b*, 178*b*
  Holmes, 163
  kinetic, 162–163
  leg
    essential tremor and, 200–201
  monosymptomatic

evaluation of, 55
movement disorders *vs.,* 163
orthostatic, 179
parkinsonism and
  differential diagnosis of, 130–131, 130*t*
PD beyond, 23–27
PD with unusual, 59–67 (*see also* multiple
      system atrophy (MSA))
postural, 162, 162*b*
resting, 162
tardive, 158
tongue
  in MSA, 102
unusual
  in PD, 59–67 (*see also* multiple system
      atrophy (MSA))
tremor associated with dystonia (TAD/
      TAWD), 136
triphosphate cyclohydrolase-1 *(GCH-1)* gene
      mutation, 201
TWSTRS. *see* Toronto Western Spasmodic
      Torticollis Rating Scale (TWSTRS)

Unified Parkinson's Disease Rating Scale
      (UPDRS-III), 32
UPDRS-III. *see* Unified Parkinson's Disease
      Rating Scale (UPDRS-III)
urinary symptoms
  in PD, 26
urinary urge/frequency
  in PD
    palliative measures for, 38*t*

variant Creutzfeldt–Jakob disease (vCJD), 208
  choreas in, 209
vascular parkinsonism, 60
  gait in, 70
vCJD. *see* variant Creutzfeldt–Jakob
      disease (vCJD)
ventral intermediate nucleus
      (VIM)/thalamus
  DBS of, 30
  in DT management, 139
vertical supranuclear gaze palsy, 72–73
VIM/thalamus. *see* ventral intermediate
      nucleus (VIM)/thalamus
VPS35 mutations
  monogenic PD and, 45*t*, 46